Dermatopathology

Diagnosis by First Impression

To Ulla, Anna, Jessica, and Sara, who let me pursue my career
while they took care of everything else. (RJB)

To Peter, who made it all possible. (CJK)

Dermatopathology
Diagnosis by First Impression

Christine J. Ko

Assistant Professor
Dermatology and Pathology
Yale University School of Medicine
New Haven
Connecticut
USA

Ronald J. Barr

Dermatopathologist
Laguna Pathology Medical Group
Laguna Beach
California;
Professor Emeritus
Dermatology and Pathology
University of California
Irvine
USA

WILEY-BLACKWELL

A John Wiley & Sons, Ltd., Publication

This edition first published 2008 © 2008 by Christine J. Ko and Ronald J. Barr

Blackwell Publishing was acquired by John Wiley & Sons in February 2007. Blackwell's publishing program has been merged with Wiley's global Scientific, Technical and Medical business to form Wiley-Blackwell.

Registered office: John Wiley & Sons Ltd, The Atrium, Southern Gate, Chichester, West Sussex, PO19 8SQ, UK

Editorial offices: 9600 Garsington Road, Oxford, OX4 2DQ, UK

The Atrium, Southern Gate, Chichester, West Sussex, PO19 8SQ, UK

111 River Street, Hoboken, NJ 07030-5774, USA

For details of our global editorial offices, for customer services and for information about how to apply for permission to reuse the copyright material in this book please see our website at www.wiley.com/wiley-blackwell

Library of Congress Cataloguing-in-Publication Data

Ko, Christine J.
    Dermatopathology : diagnosis by first impression / Christine J. Ko, Ronald J. Barr.
        p. ; cm.
    ISBN 978-1-4051-7734-4 (alk. paper)
    1. Skin—Diseases—Diagnosis—Atlases.   2. Skin—Pathophysiology—Atlases.   I. Barr, Ronald J.   II. Title.
    [DNLM: 1. Skin Diseases—diagnosis—Atlases.   2. Microscopy—Atlases. WR 17 K75d 2008]
    RL96.K6 2008
    616.5'075—dc22

2008003421

ISBN: 978-1-4051-7734-4

A catalogue record for this book is available from the British Library.

Set in 9/12pt Frutiger by Graphicraft Limited, Hong Kong
Printed in Singapore by Fabulous Printers Pte Ltd

2   2009

Contents

Preface, vi

Acknowledgments, vii

Chapter 1 Shape on Low Power, 1

Polypoid, 3

Square/rectangular, 8

Regular acanthosis, 15

Pseudoepitheliomatous hyperplasia above abscesses, 19

Proliferation downward from epidermis, 23

Central pore, 32

Palisading reactions, 36

Space with a lining, 40

Cords and tubules, 52

Papillated dermal tumor, 59

Circular dermal islands, 66

(Suggestion of) vessels, 70

Chapter 2 Top–Down, 83

Hyperkeratosis, 85

Parakeratosis, 94

Upper epidermal changes, 97

Acantholysis, 107

Eosinophilic spongiosis, 117

Subepidermal space/cleft, 124

Perivascular infiltrate, 132

Band-like upper dermal infiltrate, 137

Interface reaction, 141

Dermal material, 149

Change in fat, 162

Chapter 3 Cell Type, 175

Clear, 177

Melanocytic, 194

Spindle, 203

Giant, 216

Chapter 4 Color Blue, 225

Blue tumor, 227

Blue infiltrate, 235

Mucin and glands or ducts, 244

Mucin, 248

Chapter 5 Color Pink, 257

Pink material, 259

Pink dermis, 264

Epidermal necrosis, 267

Chapter 6 Appendix by Pattern, 273

Chapter 7 Index by Histological Category, 277

Preface

The purpose of this book is to focus on a selection of commonly tested entities, showing low- to high-power views. Major differences among diagnoses that are sometimes confused are emphasized on "Key differences" pages. As a picture is worth a thousand words, text is kept to a minimum. Since this book is not meant to replace major textbooks of dermatopathology, the atlas and the categories of differential diagnoses found in the Appendix are not comprehensive, although some entities not pictured are listed. Ultimately, the book should be used as a companion to dermatopathology textbooks and as a pictorial reference/study tool, given that this approach is utilized by the experienced dermatopathologist when constructing examination questions. Often, the major distractors are based on gestalt rather than etiology or conventional classifications. It is often the look-a-likes that prove to be the most deceptive, even though they have no obvious relationship to the correct diagnosis. This book will also be helpful to the dermatopathology novice as it introduces a simple and effective way to approach a slide.

Acknowledgments

Dr. James H. Graham, MD, master of dermatopathology and dermatology, who taught me most of what I know. (RJB)

Firstly, I would like to recognize Dr. Ronald Barr, who introduced me to the wonderful world of dermatopathology. Dermatopathology and dermatology are inextricably linked, and I also thank my other teachers at the University of California, Irvine; specifically, Dr. Gary Cole, Dr. Edward Jeffes, Dr. Vandana Nanda, Dr. Kenneth Linden, Dr. Gerald Weinstein, and Dr. Jeffrey Herten. Credit is also due to Dr. Scott Binder, an incomparable teacher and fellowship director, and to my dermatopathology colleagues at Yale (Dr. Jennifer McNiff, Dr. Earl Glusac, Dr. Rossitza Lazova, Dr. Shawn Cowper, Dr. Antonio Subtil, and Dr. Anjela Galan), who teach me things every day. Last, but not least, my family has been invaluable in supporting me through everything. (CJK)

1 Shape on Low Power

- Polypoid, 3

- Square/rectangular, 8

- Regular acanthosis, 15

- Pseudoepitheliomatous hyperplasia above abscesses, 19

- Proliferation downward from epidermis, 23

- Central pore, 32

- Palisading reactions, 36

- Space with a lining, 40

- Cords and tubules, 52

- Papillated dermal tumor, 59

- Circular dermal islands, 66

- (Suggestion of) vessels, 70

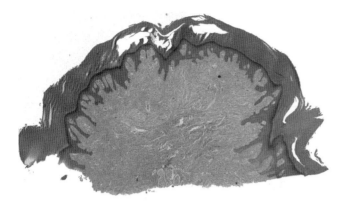

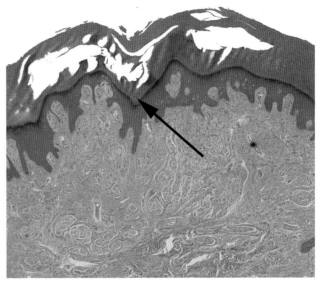

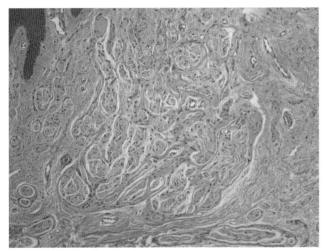

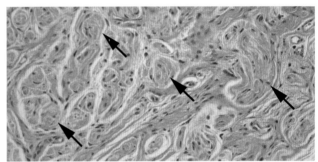

- Polypoid shape
- Acral skin [thick stratum corneum with stratum lucidum (long arrow)]
- Dermal nerve bundles (short arrows)

Accessory digit

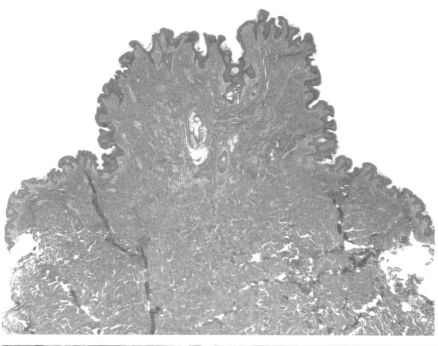

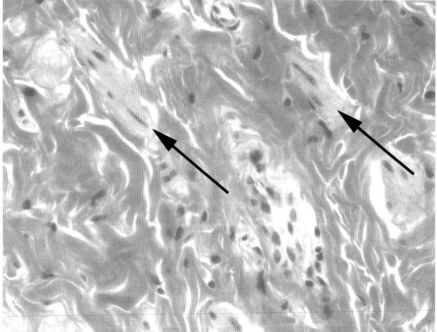

- Polypoid shape
- May see a slight invagination of surface epidermis with underlying sebaceous glands
- Surface epidermis often slightly acanthotic and hyperpigmented

- May see mammary ducts or apocrine glands deep
- Dermis with numerous smooth muscle bundles (arrows)

Accessory nipple

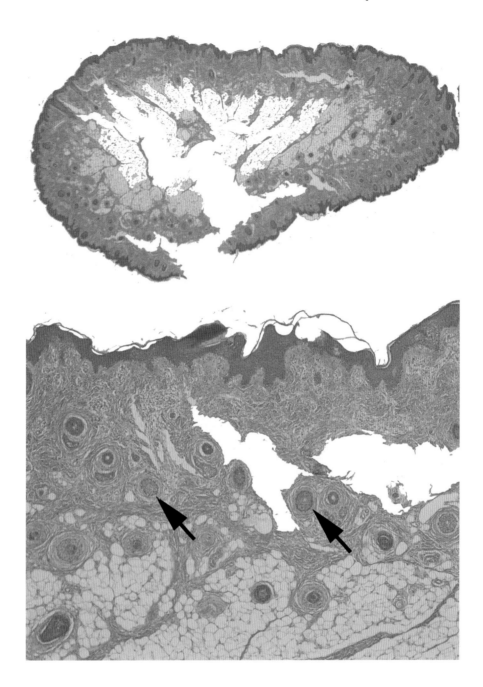

- Polypoid shape
- Thin epidermis
- Vellus hairs (arrows)
- Cartilage not always present

- Differential diagnosis of numerous vellus hairs
  - Eyelid/earlobe/sometimes facial skin
  - Vellus hair nevus

Accessory tragus

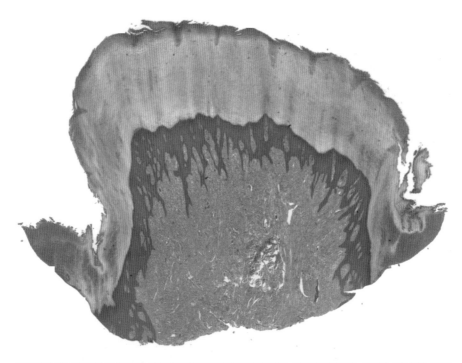

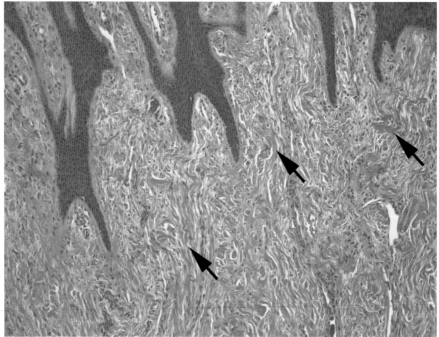

- Polypoid shape
- Acral skin
- Fibrovascular stroma [thick collagen (arrows)]

Digital fibrokeratoma

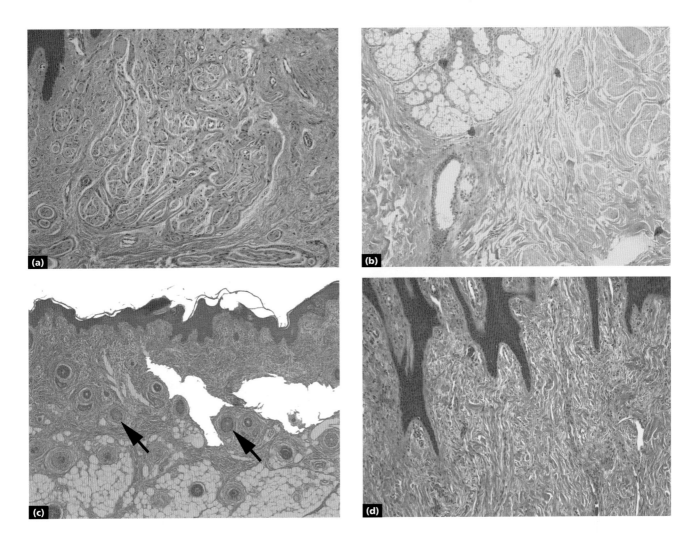

Polypoid shape

- **a** Accessory digit: nerve bundles in the dermis
- **b** Accessory nipple: sebaceous glands, mammary ducts or apocrine glands, smooth muscle bundles in the dermis
- **c** Accessory tragus: vellus hairs in the dermis
- **d** Digital fibrokeratoma: collagen in the dermis
- **Note** Other entities may also be polypoid, e.g. intradermal nevus, neurofibroma, fibrous papule

Key differences

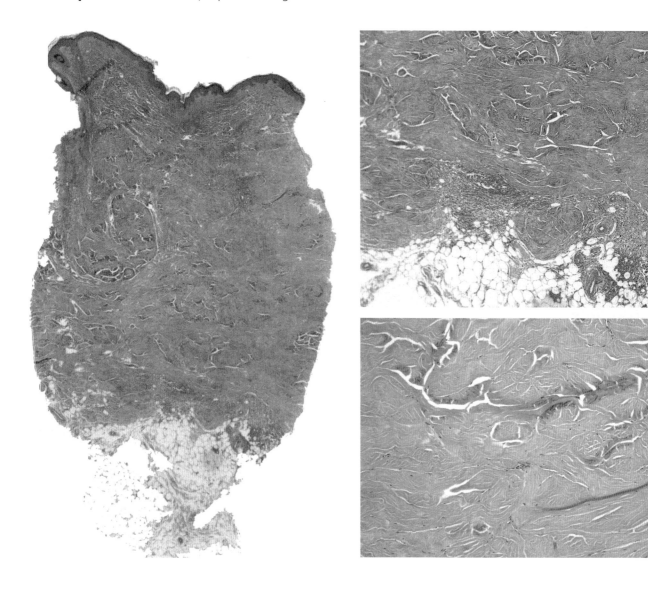

- Square/rectangular shape
- Thick, pink smudgy collagen in dermis
- Plasma cells around vessels
- Atrophic or absent adnexal structures

Morphea

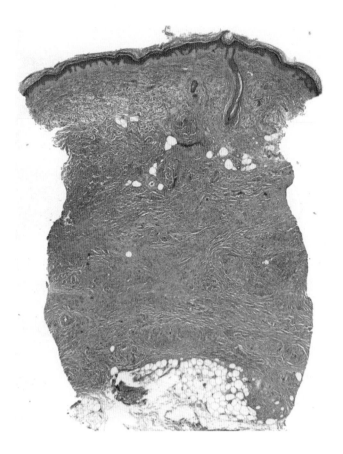

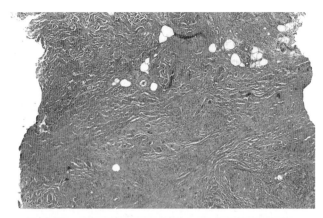

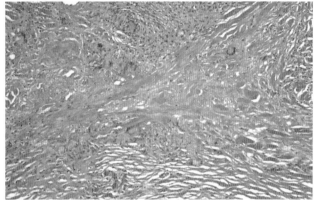

- Square/rectangular shape
- Altered, reddened collagen (necrobiosis) layered with inflammation
- Giant cells and plasma cells are prominent

Necrobiosis lipoidica

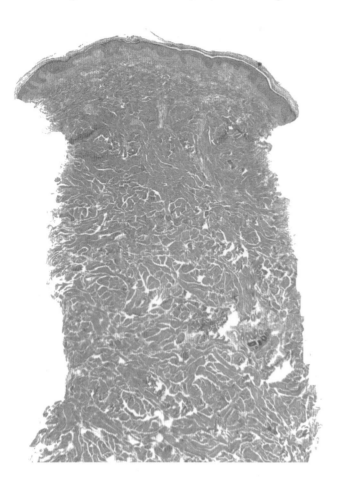

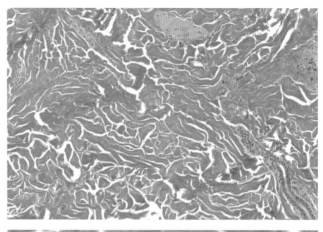

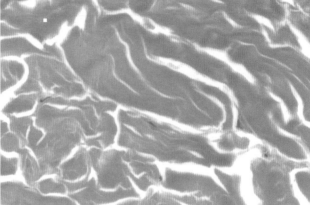

- Square/rectangular shape
- Normal-appearing collagen bundles in dermis
- No increased mucin

Normal back skin

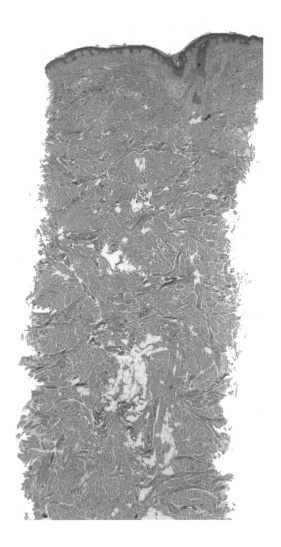

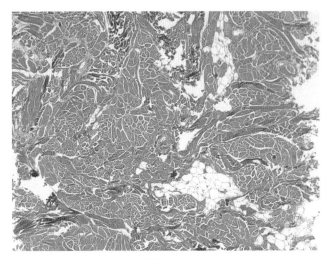

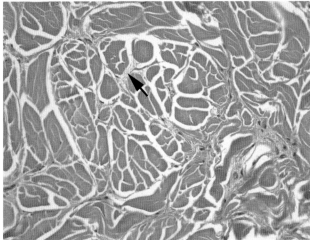

- Square/rectangular shape
- Slight widening of space between collagen due to mucin (arrow)
- No increase in fibroblasts

Scleredema

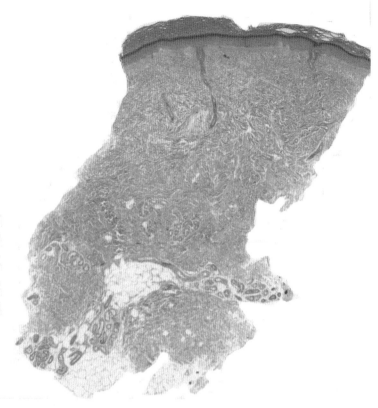

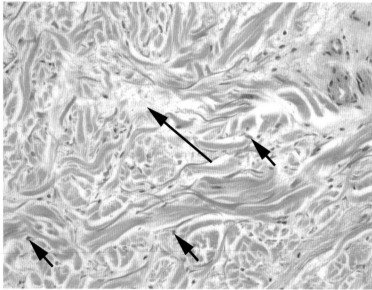

- Square/rectangular shape
- Slight widening of space between collagen due to mucin (long arrow)
- Increased fibroblasts (short arrows)

- **Note** Lichen myxedematosus is histologically similar but clinically different
- **Note** Nephrogenic systemic fibrosis may show similar findings

Scleromyxedema

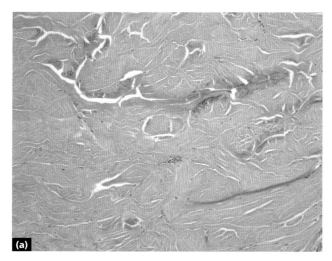

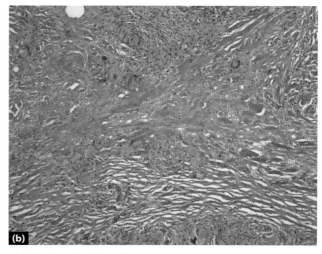

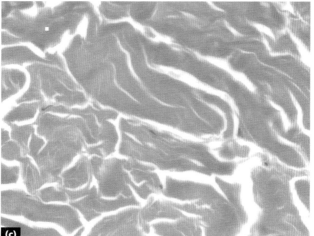

Square/rectangular shape

- **a** Morphea: thickened bundles of collagen with loss of fenestrations between collagen bundles
- **b** Necrobiosis lipoidica: reddened collagen sandwiched between layers of inflammatory cells (giant cells, plasma cells) (see also p. 39)

- **c** Normal back: normal-sized collagen bundles, no increased mucin

Key differences

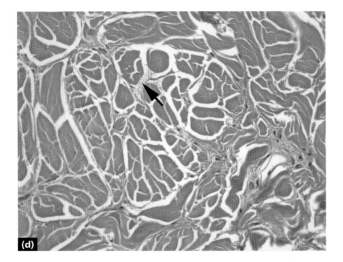

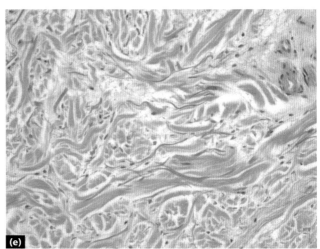

Square/rectangular shape (cont.)
- **d** Scleredema: mucin between collagen
- **e** Scleromyxedema: mucin and increased fibroblasts

Key differences

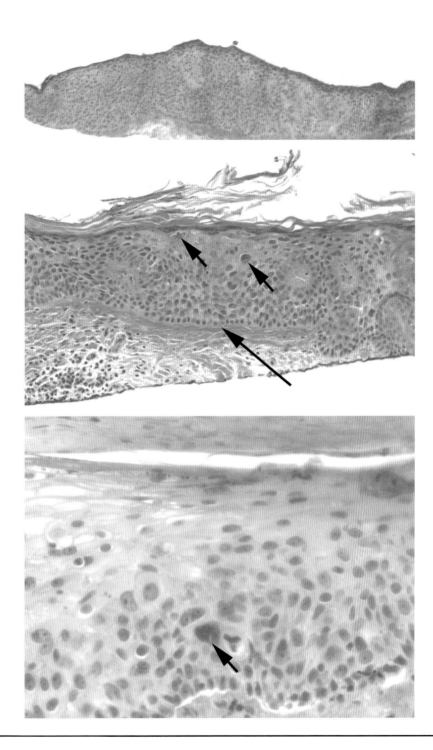

- Regular epidermal acanthosis
- Parakeratosis
- Full-thickness disorder of keratinocytes with atypical cells (short arrows) and mitoses
- Basal layer may appear normal ("eyeliner" sign) (long arrow)

Bowen's disease

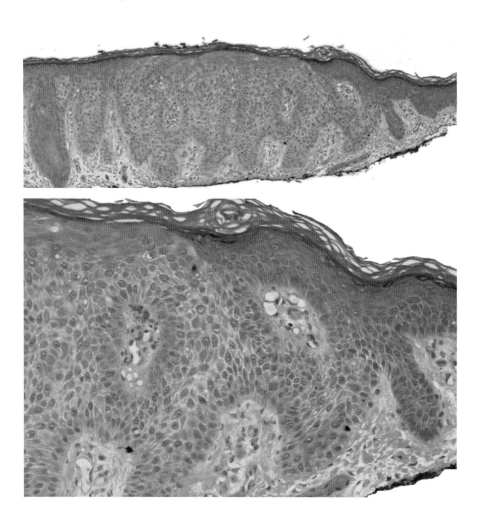

- Regular epidermal acanthosis
- Clear cells well demarcated from the normal epidermis and adnexal keratinocytes

Clear cell acanthoma

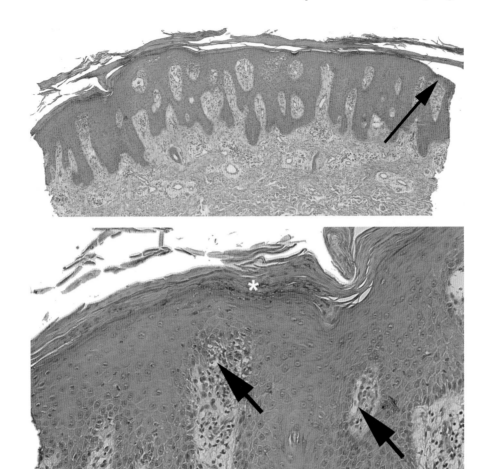

- Regular epidermal acanthosis
- Parakeratosis
- Neutrophils in stratum corneum (asterisk)
- Hypogranulosis

- Thinned suprapapillary plates (long arrow)
- Dilated vessels in papillary dermis (short arrows)

Psoriasis

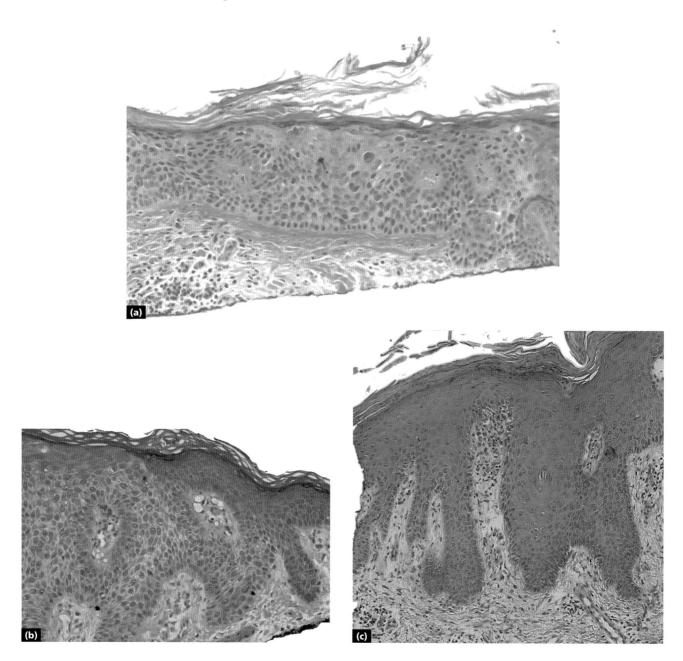

Regular epidermal acanthosis

- **a** Bowen's disease: disordered keratinocytes and atypical mitoses
- **b** Clear cell acanthoma: pale/clear keratinocytes well demarcated from normal epidermis

- **c** Psoriasis: confluent parakeratosis above thickened epidermis, neutrophils in stratum corneum, normal keratinocytes, thin suprapapillary plates, dilated vessels

Key differences

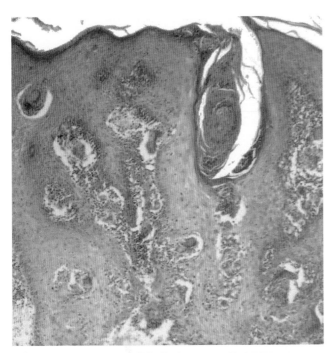
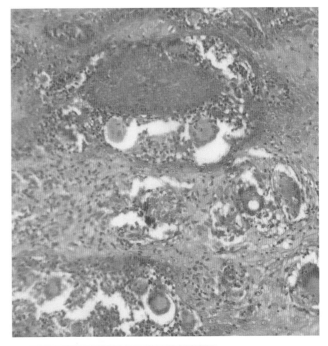
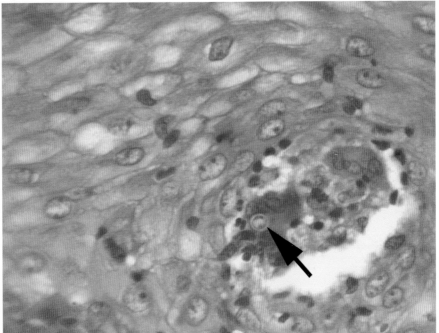

- Pseudoepitheliomatous hyperplasia above abscesses
- Yeast forms (arrow) that classically show broad-based budding

Blastomycosis

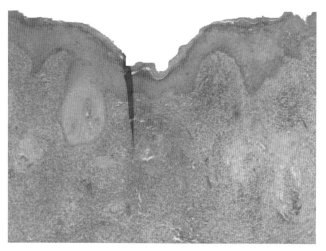

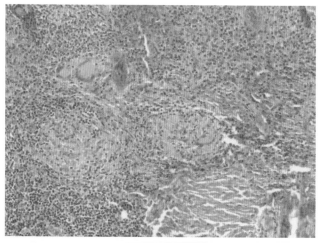

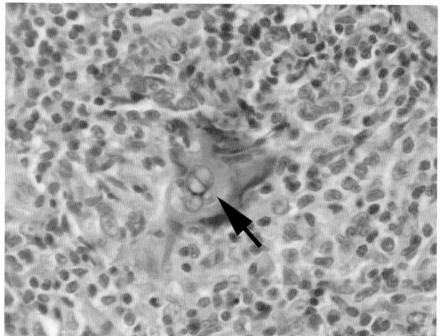

- Pseudoepitheliomatous hyperplasia above abscesses
- Brown-colored septate rounded "hot cross buns"
  (Medlar bodies, sclerotic bodies, copper pennies) (arrow)

Chromomycosis

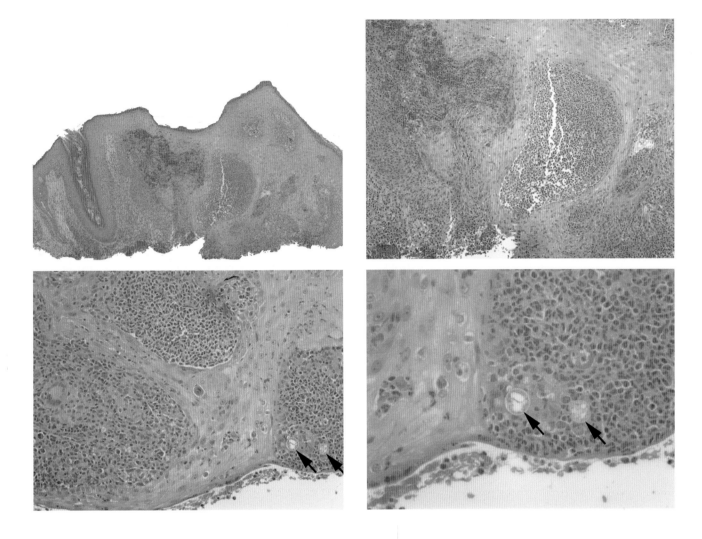

- Pseudoepitheliomatous hyperplasia above abscesses
- Large (80–200 µm) spherules containing endospores
  (arrows)

Coccidioidomycosis

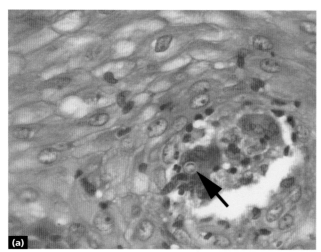

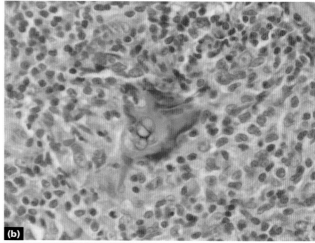

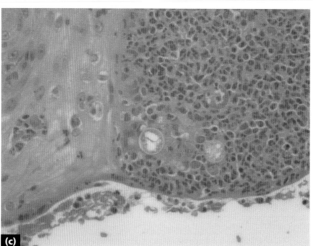

Pseudoepitheliomatous hyperplasia above abscesses
- **a** Blastomycosis: 8–30 μm yeast form (arrow)
- **b** Chromomycosis: 5–12 μm Medlar bodies
- **c** Coccidioidomycosis: 80–200 μm spherules with endospores

- **Note** Paracoccidioidomycosis (6–60 μm mariner's wheel; an uncommon infection in the United States), sporotrichosis (organisms usually not evident in biopsies), and tuberculosis verrucosa cutis may also show this pattern

Key differences

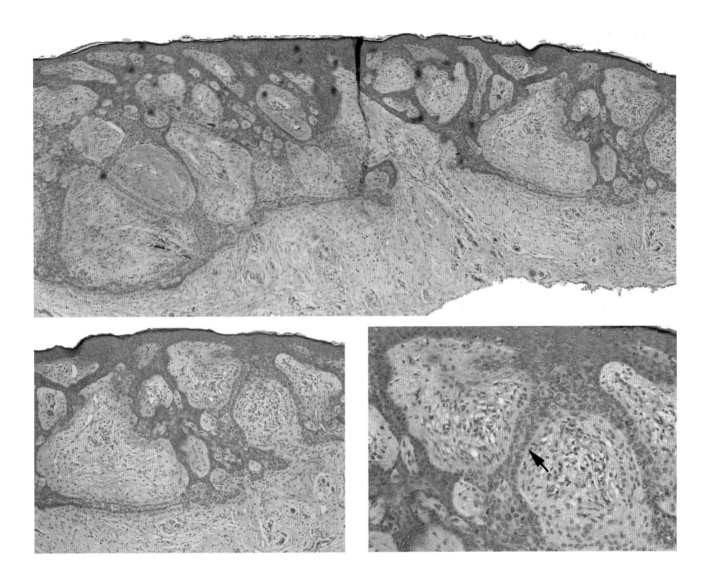

- Proliferation downward from epidermis
- Strands of basaloid cells in a fibrovascular stroma often emanating from strands of squamous epithelium
- Some hints of palisading of cells (arrow)

Fibroepithelioma of Pinkus

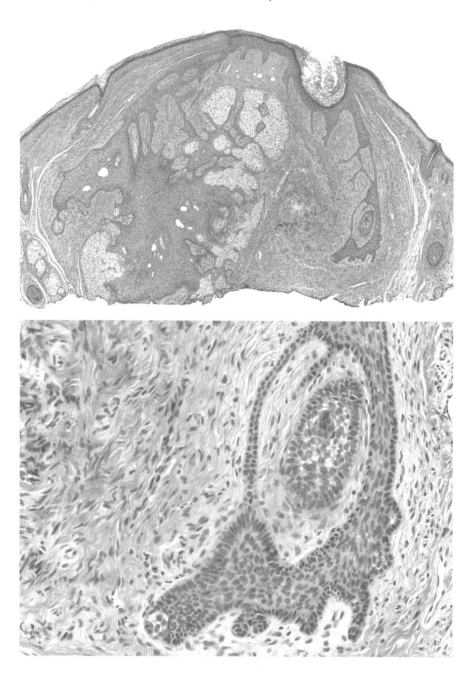

- Proliferation downward from epidermis
- Fibrotic stroma adjacent to the hair follicle has reticulated strands of epithelium
- This entity has overlap with trichodiscoma (some consider these a spectrum of the same entity)

Fibrofolliculoma

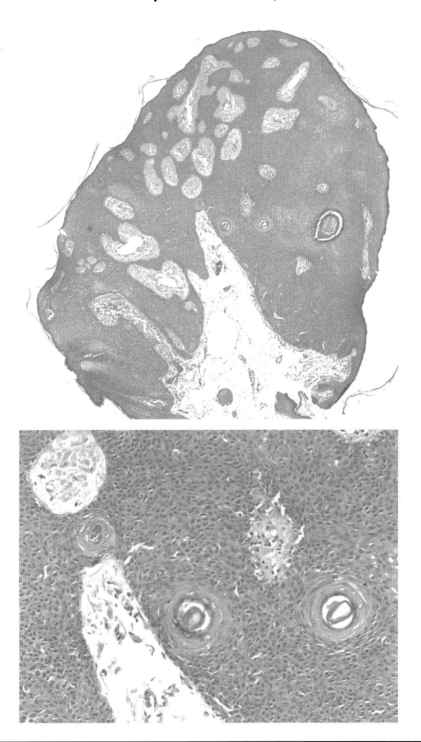

- Proliferation downward from epidermis
- Normal-appearing keratinocytes with some arranged in squamous eddies causing intraepithelial fenestrations

Inverted follicular keratosis

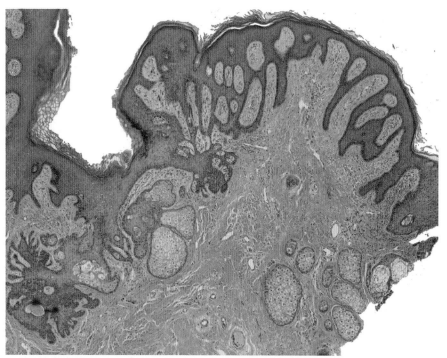

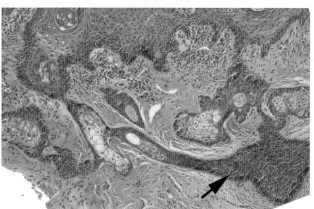

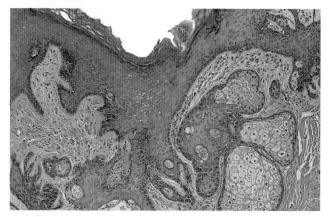

- Proliferation downward from epidermis
- Sebaceous glands, basaloid proliferations (arrow) connect to the epidermis
- Apocrine glands may be seen deep
- Absent terminal hairs in mature stage

Acanthosis, papillomatosis, hyperkeratosis

Nevus sebaceus of Jadassohn

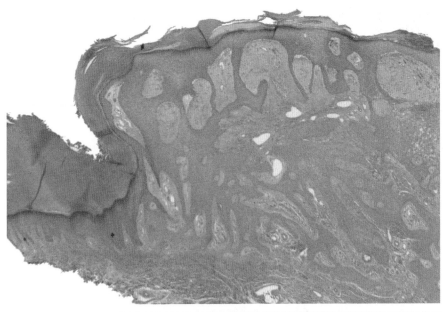

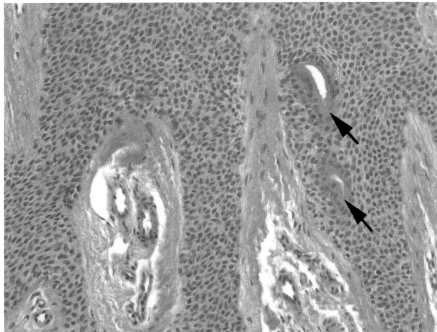

- Proliferation downward from epidermis
- Uniform blue cells with interspersed ducts (arrows)
- Fibrotic or hyalinized stroma with dilated vessels

Poroma

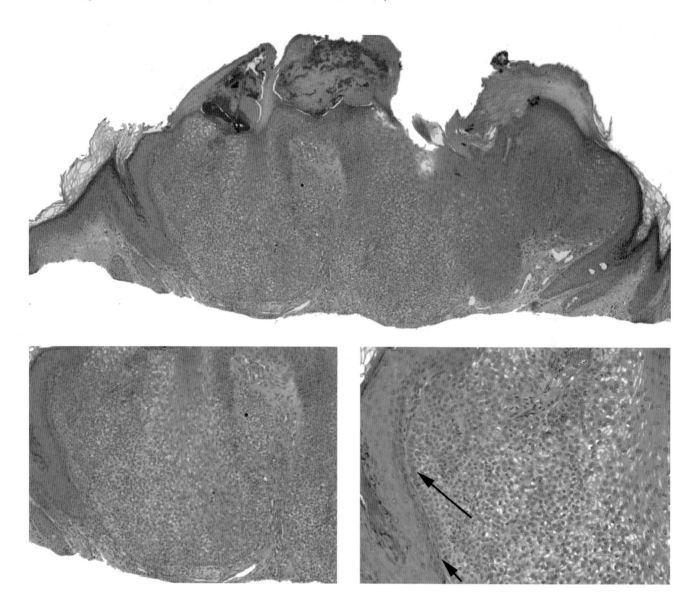

- Proliferation downward from epidermis
- Proliferation composed of pale/clear cells
- Peripheral palisading (long arrow) with thickened basement membrane (short arrow)

Trichilemmoma

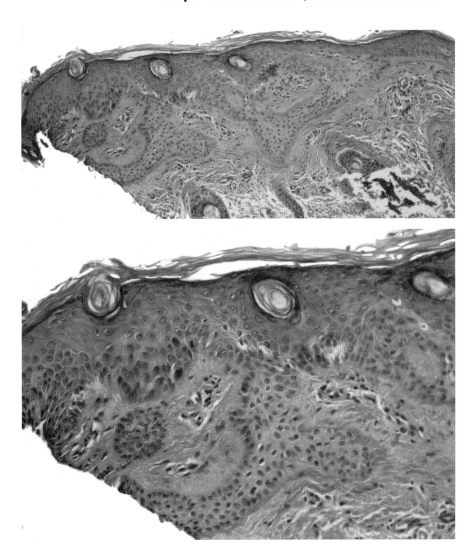

- Proliferation downward from epidermis
- Pale cells in columns with "windows" of dermis in between
- Peripheral palisading

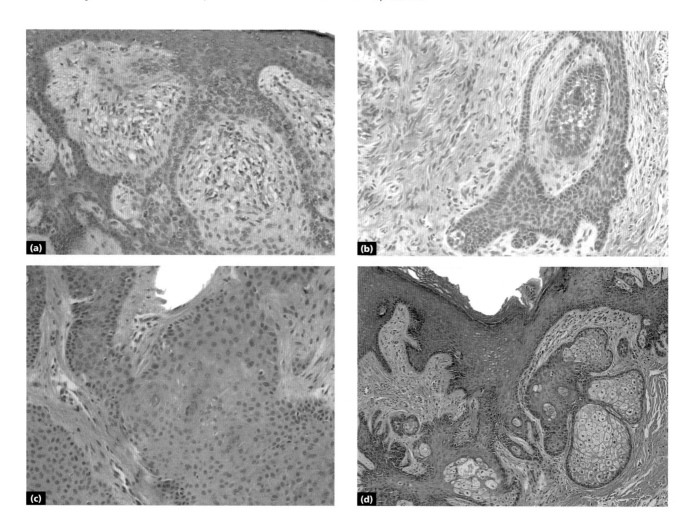

Proliferation downward from epidermis

- **a** Fibroepithelioma of Pinkus: strands of basaloid epithelium in fibrovascular stroma
- **b** Fibrofolliculoma: hair follicle with adjacent fibrotic stroma and reticulated epithelium
- **c** Inverted follicular keratosis: squamous eddies
- **d** Nevus sebaceus of Jadassohn: proliferation of epidermis connecting to sebaceous lobules and basaloid proliferations

Key differences

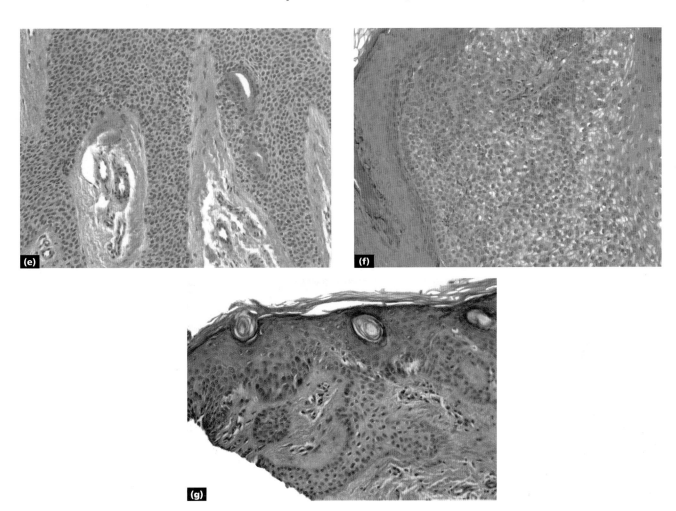

Proliferation downward from epidermis (cont.)

- **e** Poroma: uniform blue cells with interspersed ducts
- **f** Trichilemmoma: pale/clear keratinocytes with peripheral palisading and thickened basement membrane
- **g** Tumor of the follicular infundibulum: pale cells in columns with "windows" of dermis in between

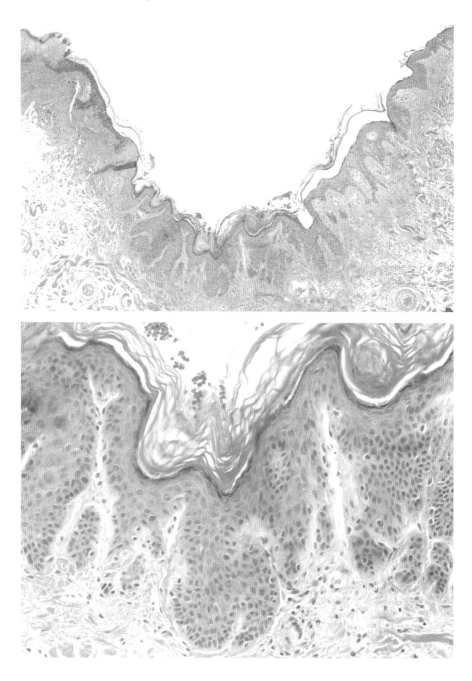

- Central pore
- Invaginated epidermis is acanthotic

Dilated pore of Winer

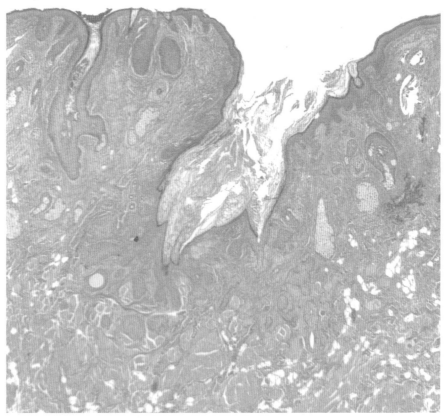

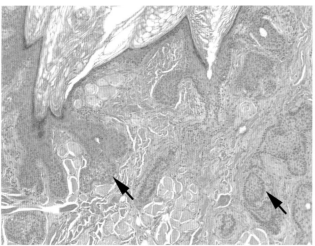 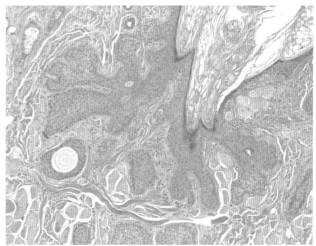

- Central pore
- Invaginated epidermis is acanthotic and has areas resembling outer root sheath with peripheral palisading around slightly pale cells (arrows)

Pilar sheath acanthoma

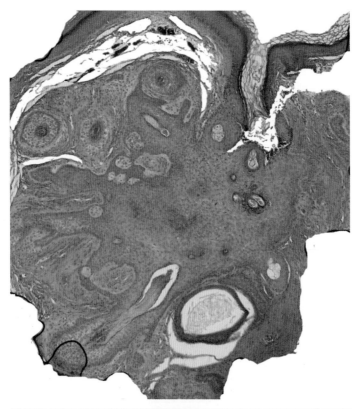

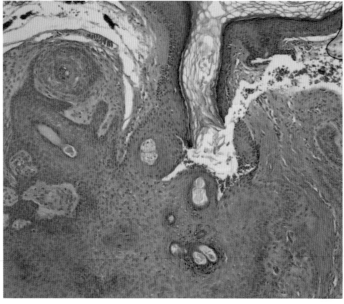

- Central pore
- Invaginated epidermis connects to a primary hair follicle
- Multiple secondary hair follicles radiating away from
  the central follicle

Trichofolliculoma

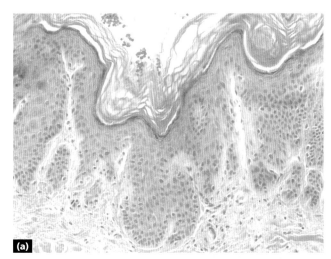

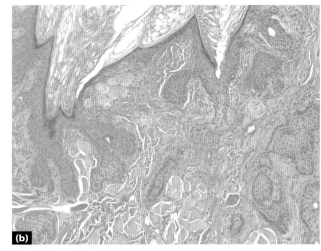

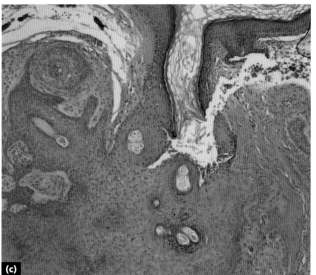

Central pore

- **a** Dilated pore of Winer: acanthotic epidermis
- **b** Pilar sheath acanthoma: epidermal acanthosis and areas resembling outer root sheath
- **c** Trichofolliculoma: primary follicle and surrounding secondary follicles

Key differences

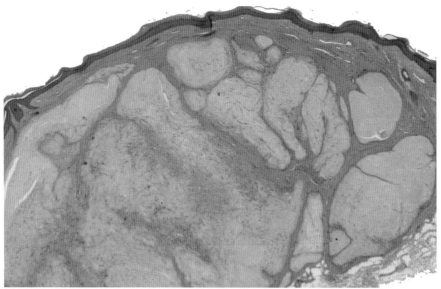

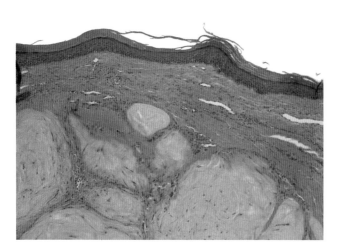
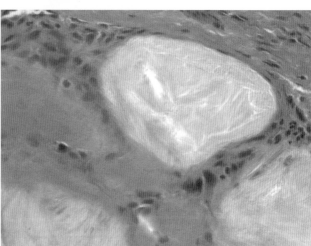

- Palisading of histiocytes around amorphous
  white–gray substance with a feathery edge

Gout

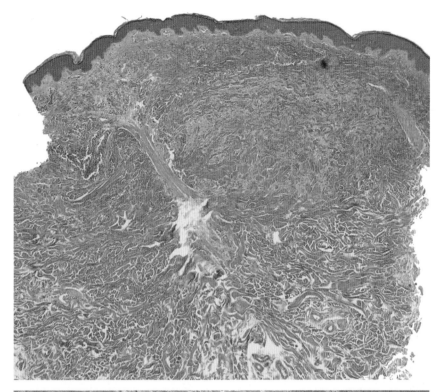

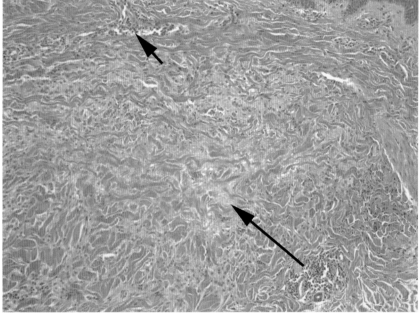

- Palisading of histiocytes around altered collagen, basophilic mucin (long arrow)
- Lymphocytes around vessels (short arrow)

Granuloma annulare

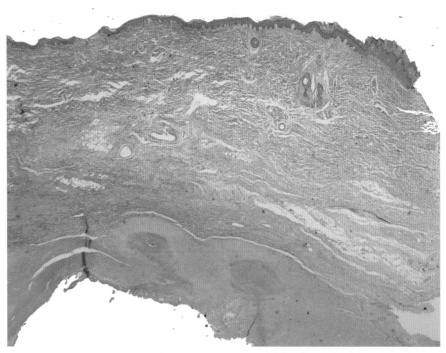

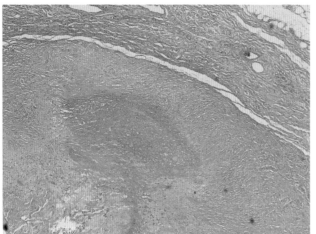
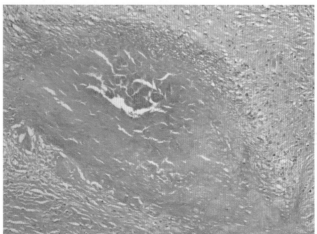

- Palisading of histiocytes around central pink fibrin
- The reaction is often deep

Rheumatoid nodule

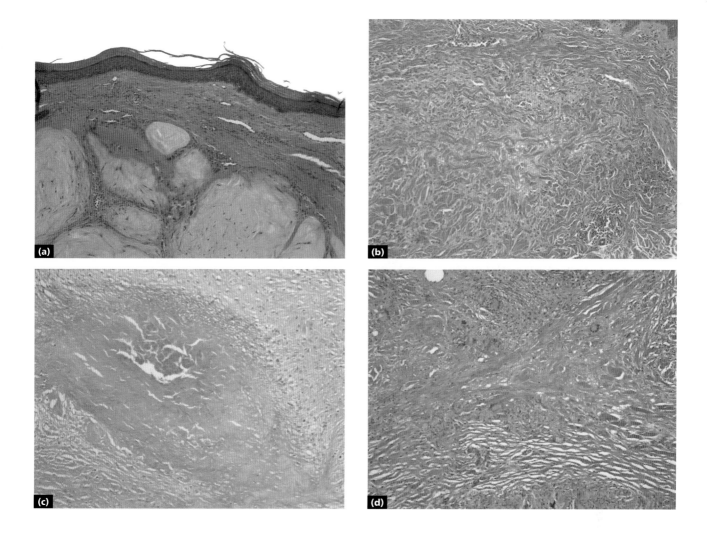

Palisading reactions

- **a** Gout: central white–gray feathery material
- **b** Granuloma annulare: central altered collagen interspersed with blue mucin
- **c** Rheumatoid nodule: central pink fibrin
- **d** Necrobiosis lipoidica: altered collagen surrounded by giant cells, plasma cells (see also pp. 9 and 13)

Key differences

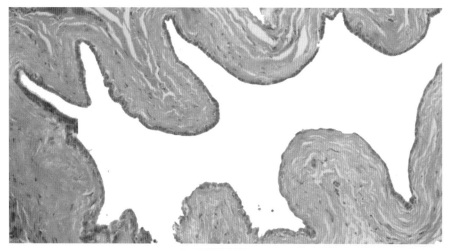

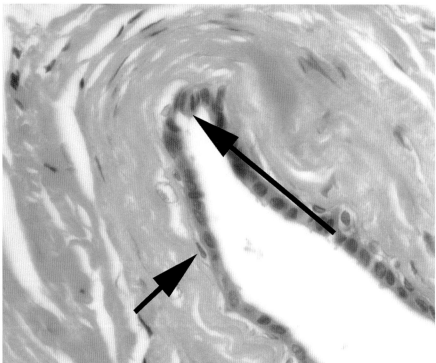

- Space with a lining
- Lining composed of an inner layer of cells with decapitation secretion (long arrow) and a compressed layer of myoepithelial cells (short arrow)

Apocrine hidrocystoma

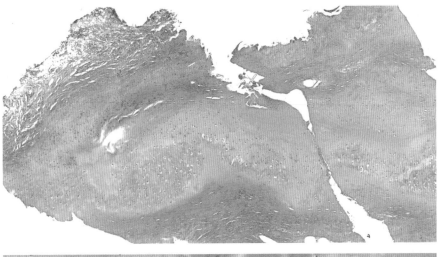

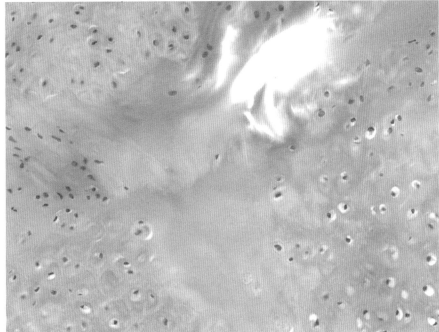

- Space with a lining
- "Lining" is not a true epithelial layer but is cartilage
- Centrally, there is degeneration of cartilage

Auricular pseudocyst

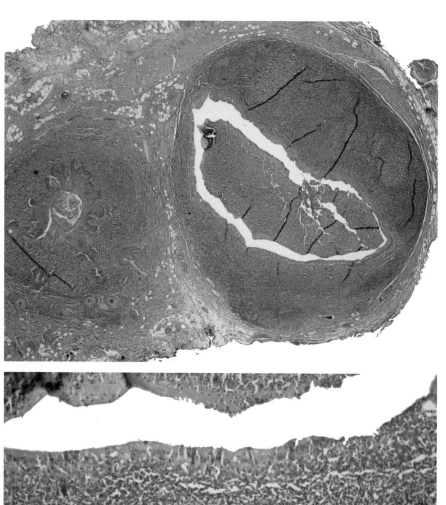

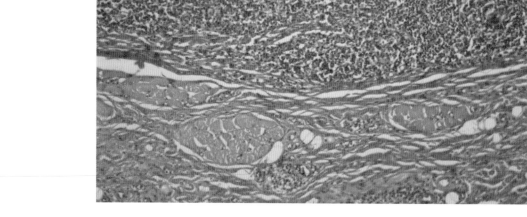

- Space with a lining
- Lining composed of squamous or sometimes cuboidal/
  columnar epithelium often with squamous metaplasia
- Prominent lymphoid follicles in wall

Branchial cleft cyst

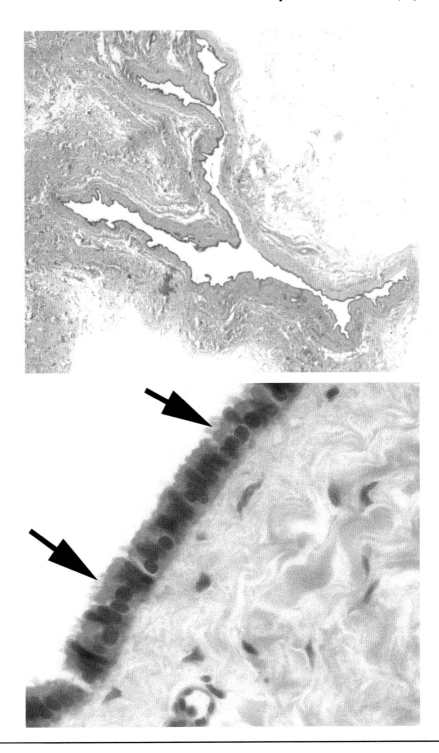

- Space with a lining
- Lining composed of cuboidal/columnar epithelium with cilia
  (arrows)

Cutaneous ciliated cyst

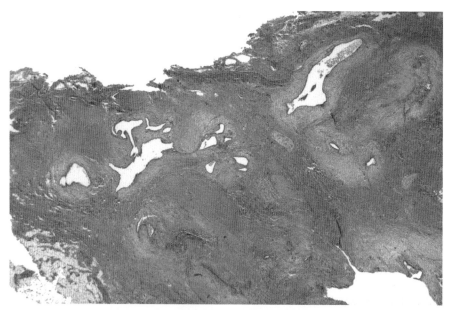

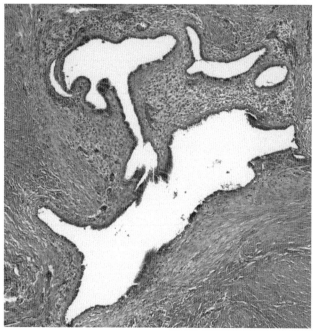

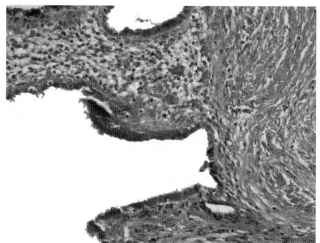

- Space with a lining
- Spaces embedded in a fibrovascular stroma (endometrial stroma)
- Lining composed of crowded blue cells
- Hemosiderin deposits common in stroma

Cutaneous endometriosis

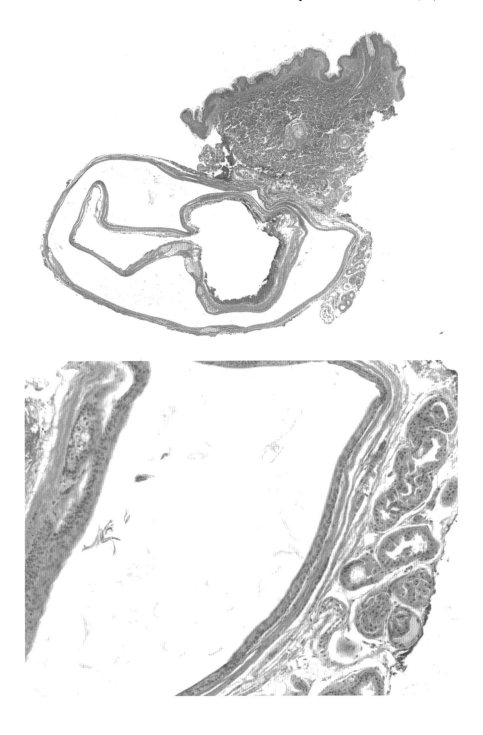

- Space with a lining
- Lining composed of squamous epithelium
- Walls contain adnexal structures

Dermoid cyst

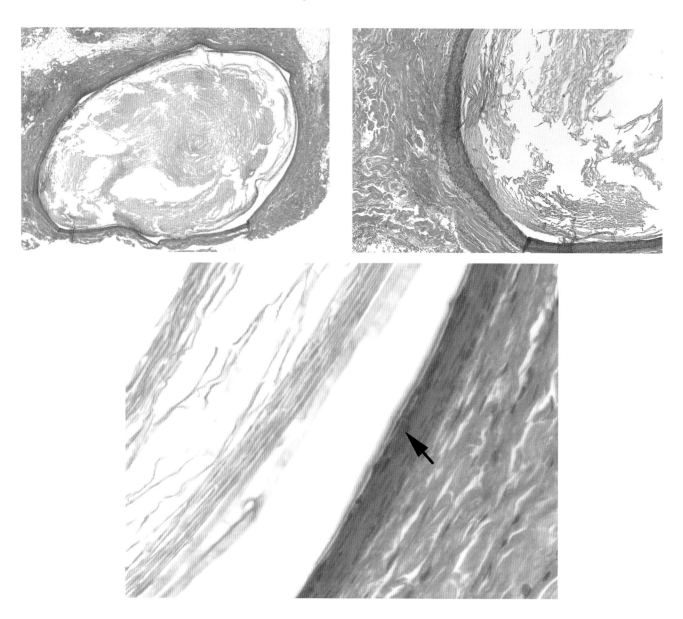

- Space with a lining
- Lining composed of squamous epithelium with a granular layer (arrow)
- Cyst contents composed of flakes of keratin

Epidermal inclusion cyst

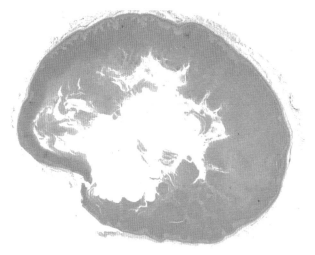

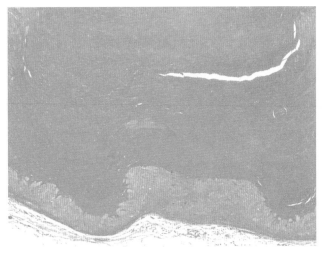

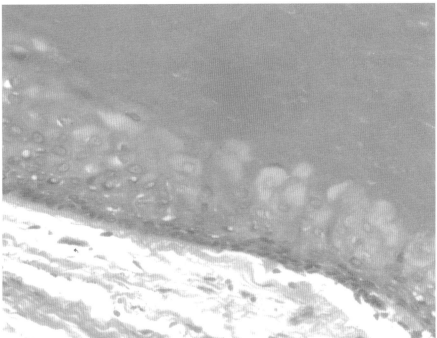

- Space with a lining
- Lining composed of squamous epithelium without
  a granular layer
- Cyst contents composed of dense pink keratin

Pilar cyst

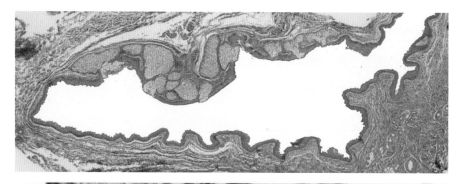

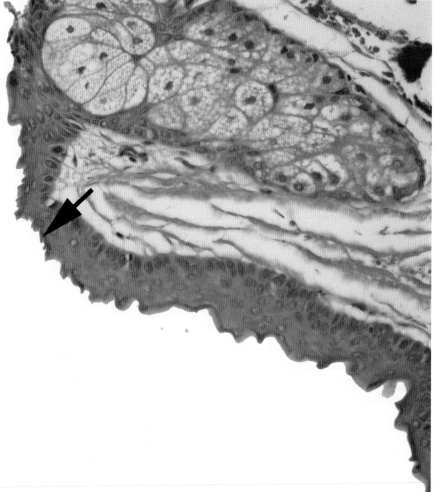

- Space with a lining
- Lining composed of layered epithelium with a bright pink crenulated keratin (arrow)
- Sebaceous glands in wall

Steatocystoma

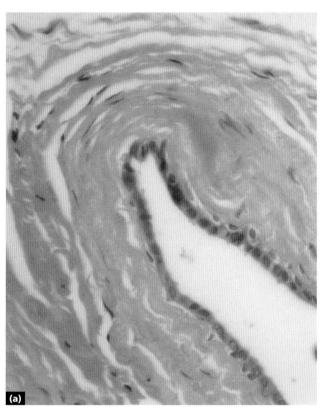

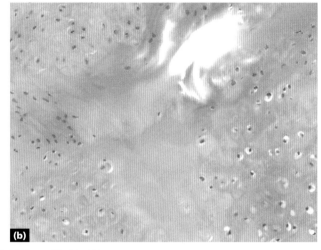

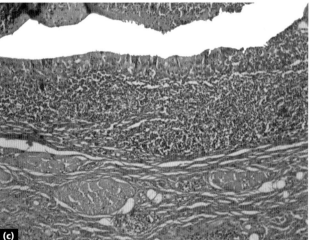

Space with a lining

- **a** Apocrine hidrocystoma: decapitation secretion
- **b** Auricular pseudocyst: degeneration surrounded by cartilage
- **c** Branchial cleft cyst: prominent lymphoid follicles in wall

Key differences

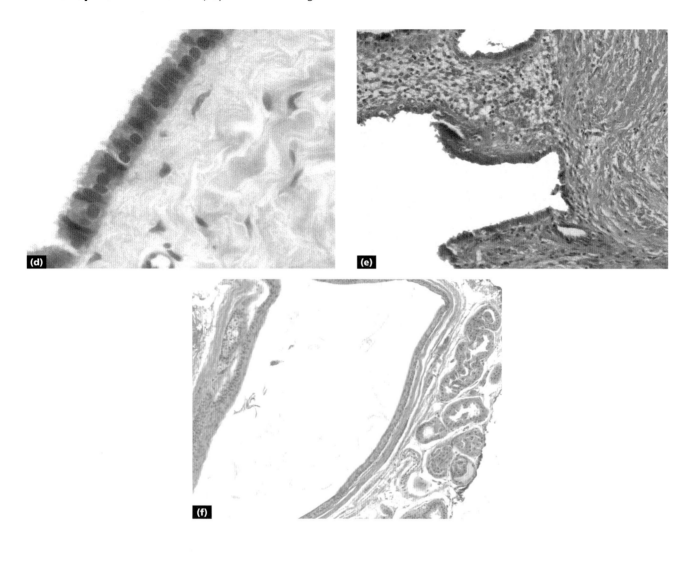

Space with a lining (cont.)

- **d** Cutaneous ciliated cyst: columnar epithelium with cilia; no structures in wall
- **e** Cutaneous endometriosis: fibrovascular stroma with glands
- **f** Dermoid cyst: sebaceous glands and other adnexal structures in wall

Key differences

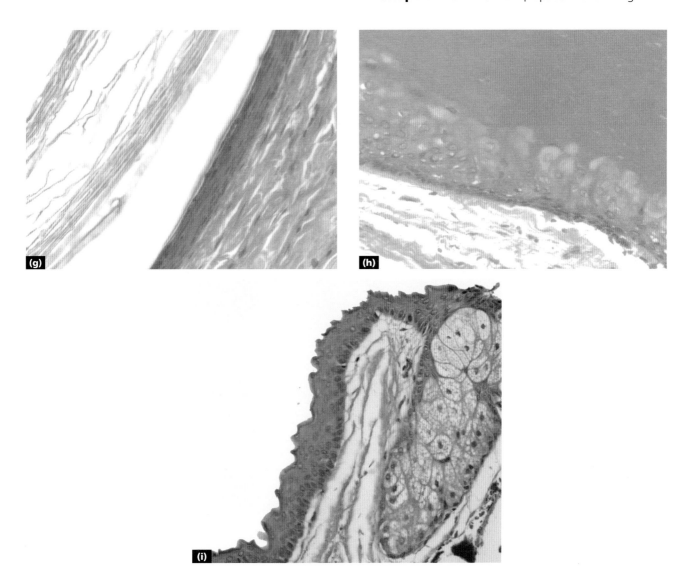

Space with a lining (cont.)

- **g** Epidermal inclusion cyst: epithelium with granular layer, flakes of keratin in center
- **h** Pilar cyst: epithelium without granular layer, dense keratin in center
- **i** Steatocystoma: crenulated keratin lining the cyst; sebaceous glands in wall

- **Note** Bronchogenic cysts are uncommon, and are diagnosed by clinical history and the presence of columnar epithelium +/– cilia, +/– cartilage in the wall; venous lakes are common and are composed of flattened endothelial cells with erythrocytes in the space

Key differences

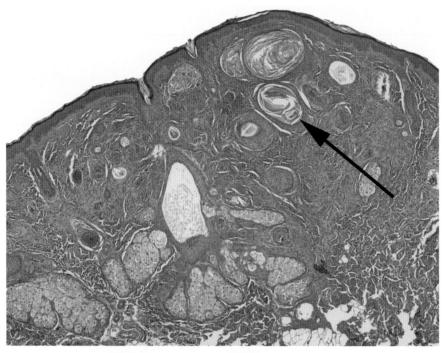

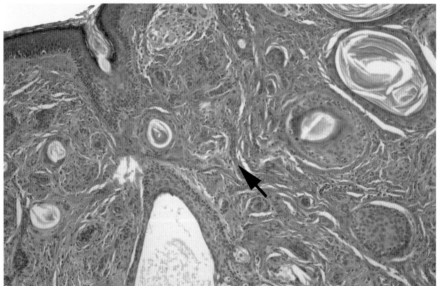

- Cords and tubules in dermis
- Numerous horn cysts (long arrow) in fibrotic stroma
- Tubules of two-layered epithelium (short arrow)
- Calcification often present
- Confined to dermis

Desmoplastic trichoepithelioma

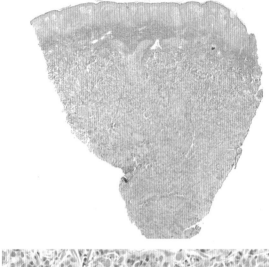

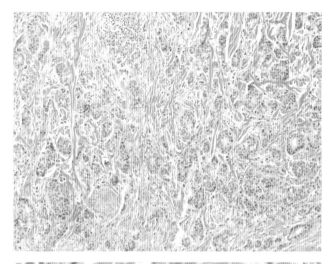

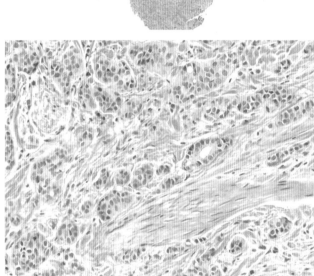

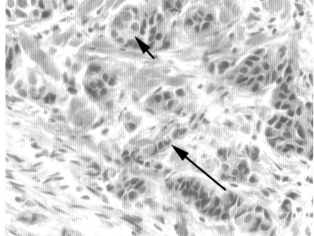

- Cords and tubules in dermis
- Tubules of single-layered ("Indian filing", long arrow) and multilayered epithelium
- Some cells forming gland-like structures (short arrow)

- Other metastatic carcinomas may look like this – need clinical history; immunohistochemistry may be helpful

Metastatic breast carcinoma

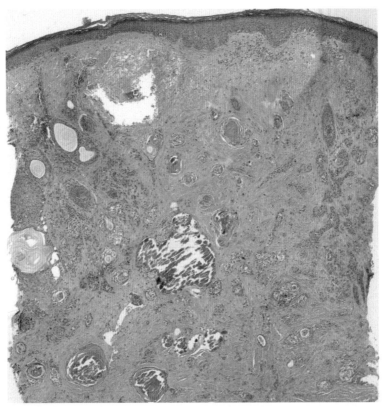

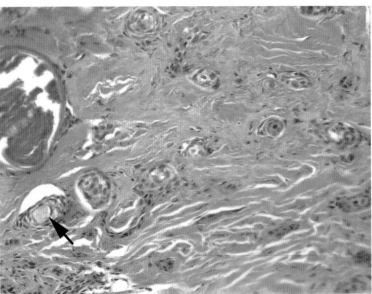

- Cords and tubules in dermis
- Tubules of epithelium connect to islands of epithelium
  with duct-like spaces (arrow)
- Deeply infiltrative (fills dermis)
- Perineural involvement

Microcystic adnexal carcinoma

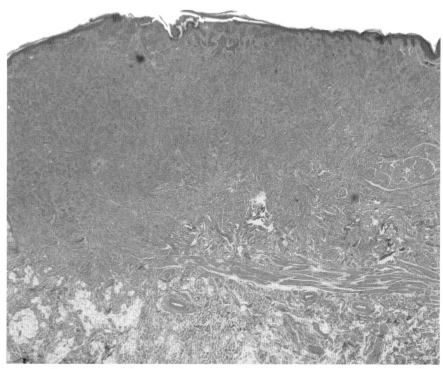

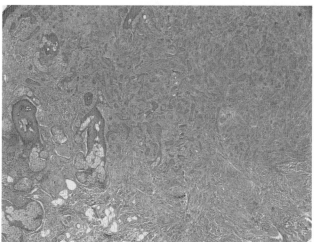
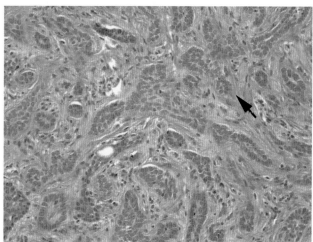

- Cords and tubules in dermis
- Cords of epithelium composed of basaloid cells with hints
  of peripheral palisading
- New collagen forming around islands (arrow)
- Deeply infiltrative

Morpheaform basal cell carcinoma

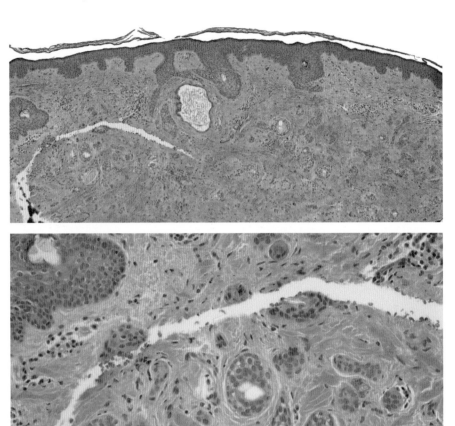

- Cords and tubules in dermis
- Restricted to upper dermis
- "Tadpoles" of epithelium with duct-like structures in heads (arrow)

- Darker cells at periphery, clear cells in center
- Eosinophilic cuticle lining lumina
- No horn cysts

Syringoma

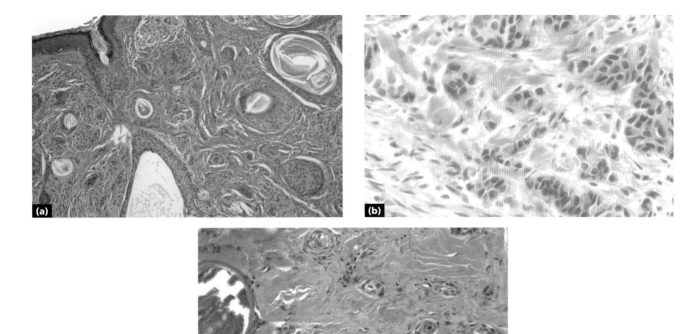

Cords and tubules

- **a** Desmoplastic trichoepithelioma: horn cysts, no clear cells, circular areas of epithelium surround keratin
- **b** Metastatic breast carcinoma: single filing of atypical cells, deeply infiltrative
- **c** Microcystic adnexal carcinoma: like syringoma with tadpole-like structures but deeply infiltrative, perineural involvement

Key differences

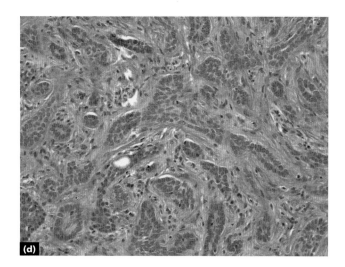

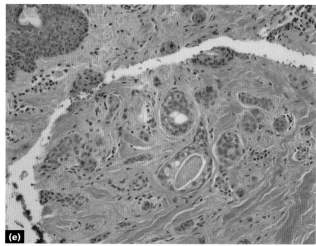

Cords and tubules (cont.)

- **d** Morpheaform basal cell carcinoma: infiltrative cords of
  basaloid cells with hints of peripheral palisading; may have
  some duct-like structures (but fewer than **c**)
- **e** Syringoma: superficial tadpoles with clear cells

Key differences

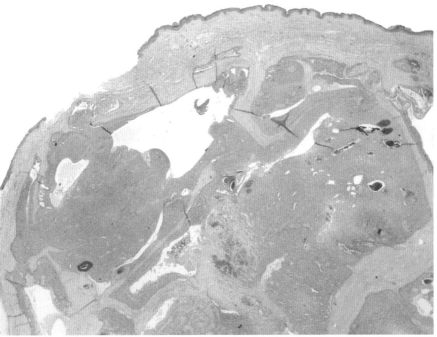

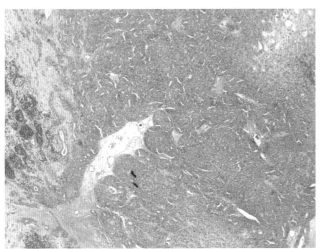
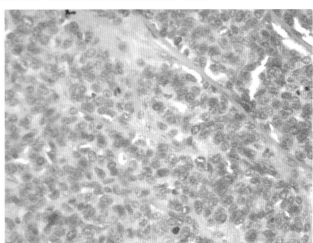

- Papillated dermal tumor
- Disordered layers of epithelium in large papillations with some tubules
- Variable cytological atypia and mitotic figures
- Acral location

Aggressive digital papillary adenocarcinoma

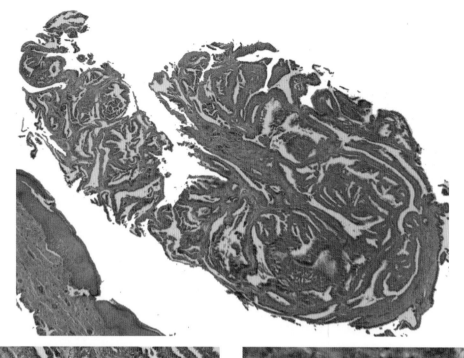

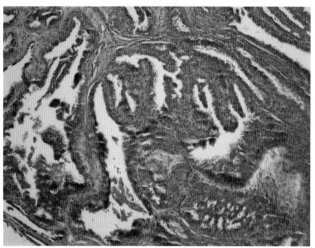
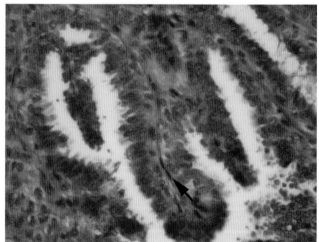

- Papillated dermal tumor
- Finger-like projections have cores of collagen/fibroblasts
  (arrow)
- No connection to epidermis

Hidradenoma papilliferum

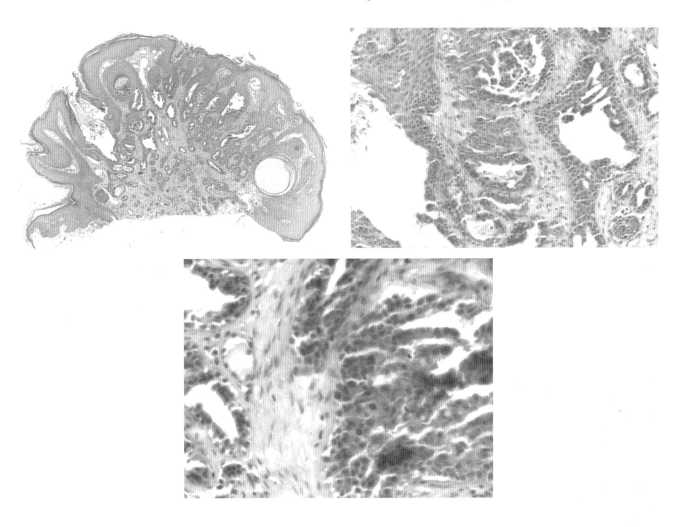

- Papillated dermal tumor
- Islands of epithelium with papillated projections
- With or without epidermal connection

Papillary eccrine adenoma

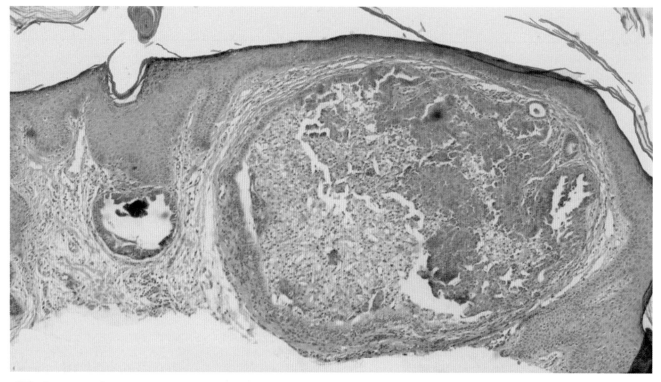

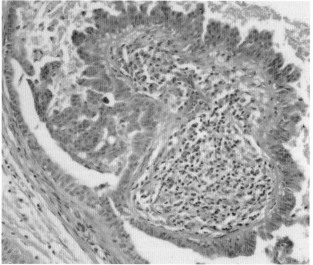
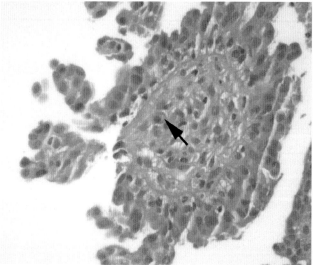

- Papillated dermal tumor
- Papillations contain numerous plasma cells (arrow)
- Tumor often connected to epidermis

Syringocystadenoma papilliferum

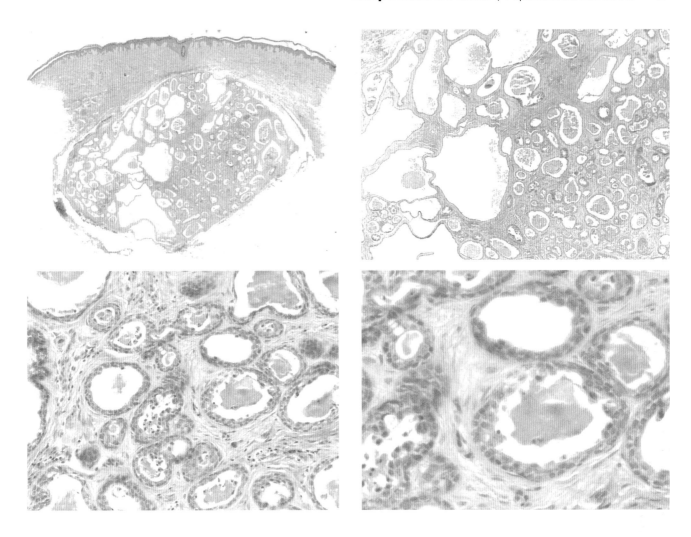

- Papillated dermal tumor
- Evidence of decapitation secretion
- Overlaps with papillary eccrine adenoma

Tubular apocrine adenoma

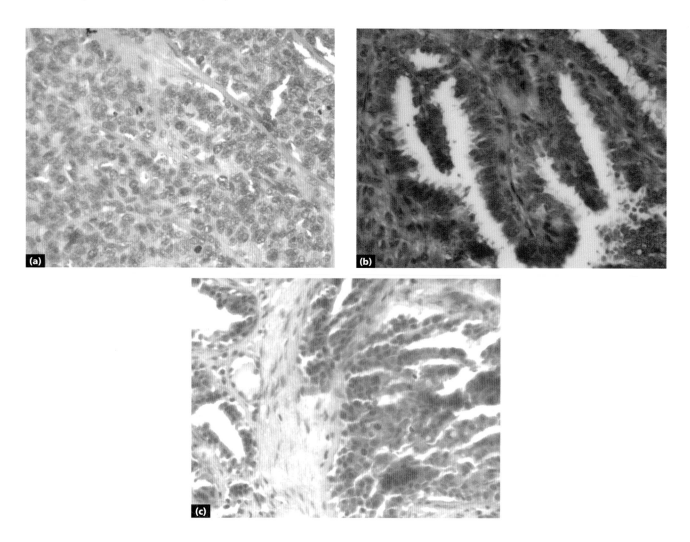

Papillated dermal tumor

- **a** Aggressive digital papillary adenocarcinoma: large tumor, atypical cells, and mitoses piled up
- **b** Hidradenoma papilliferum: thin papillations with fibrovascular cores

- **c** Papillary eccrine adenoma: islands of epithelium with papillated areas

Key differences

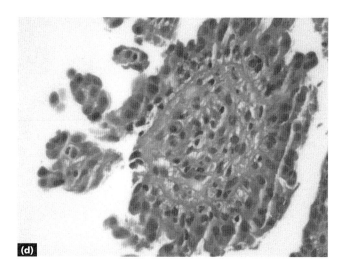

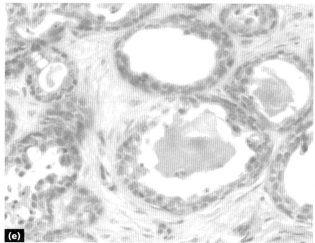

Papillated dermal tumor (cont.)

- **d** Syringocystadenoma papilliferum: broad papillations with plasma cells in cores
- **e** Tubular apocrine adenoma: decapitation secretion and papillations within islands

Key differences

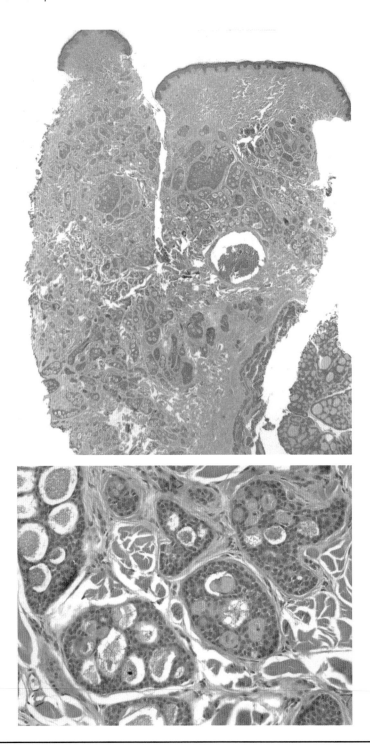

- Circular dermal islands
- Islands contain basaloid cells with a cribriform pattern of duct-like spaces filled with amorphous material

Adenoid cystic carcinoma

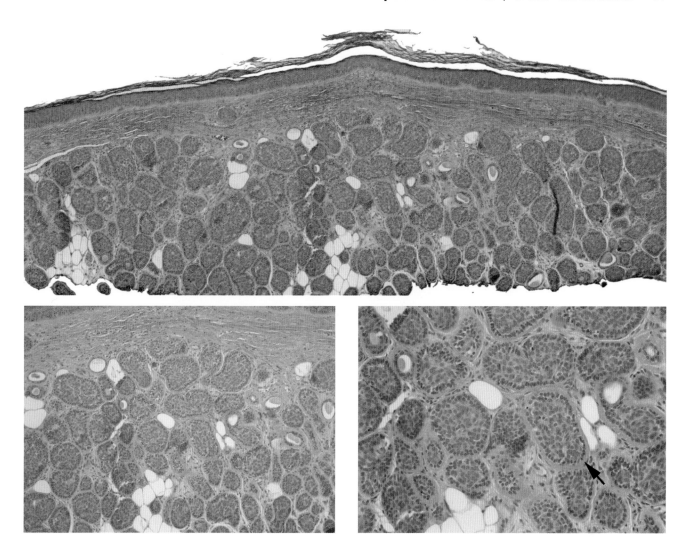

- Circular dermal islands
- Islands contain basaloid cells surrounded by a thick pink basement membrane (arrow)
- Islands arranged like a "jigsaw puzzle"

Cylindroma

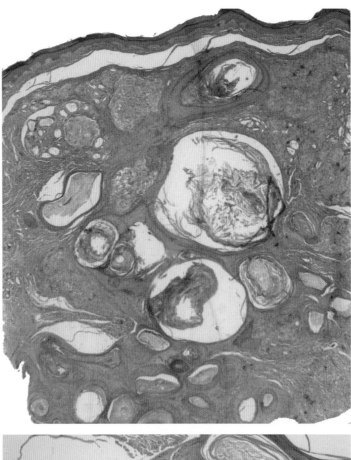

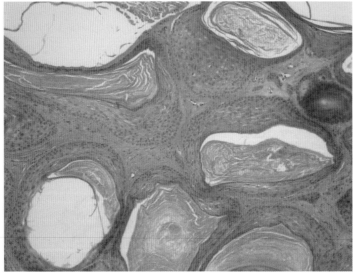

- Circular dermal islands
- Islands of epithelium with central flaky keratin (horn cysts)

Trichoadenoma

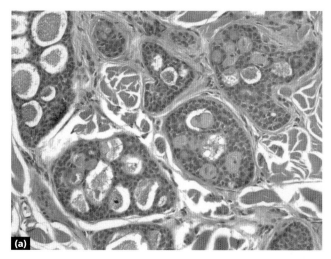

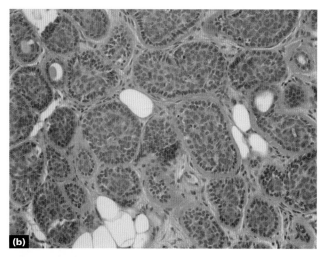

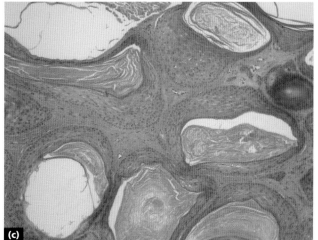

Circular dermal islands

- **a** Adenoid cystic carcinoma: cribriform pattern of duct-like structures
- **b** Cylindroma: puzzle-like arrangement, thick/pink basement membrane
- **c** Trichoadenoma: numerous horn cysts

Key differences

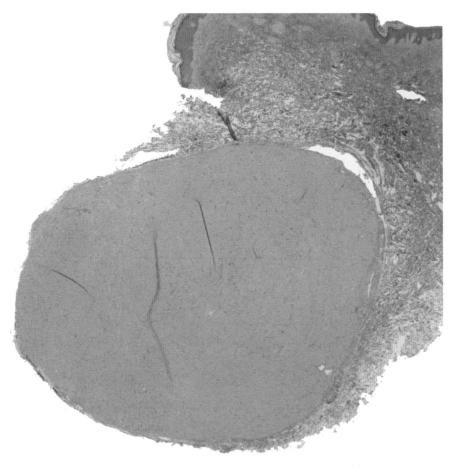

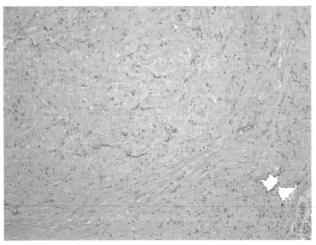

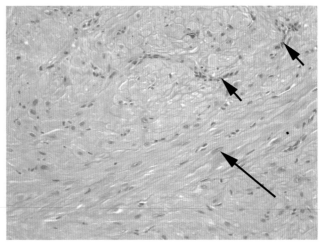

- (Suggestion of) vessels
- Circular pink mass in dermis
- Scar-like appearance

- Mass composed of smooth muscle cells (cigar-shaped nuclei, long arrows) with compressed vessels (short arrows) (sometimes dilated)

Angioleiomyoma

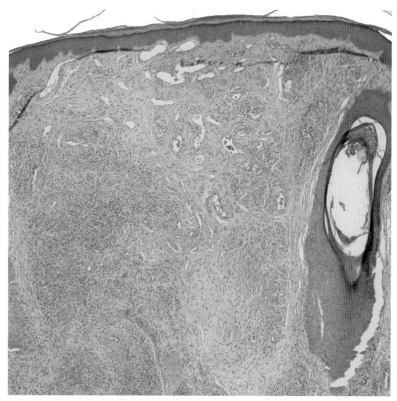

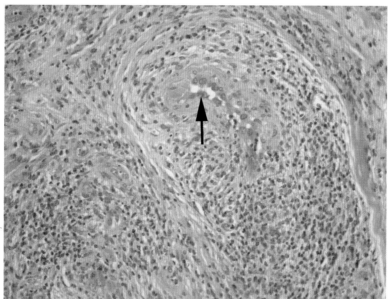

- (Suggestion of) vessels
- Numerous vessels with epithelioid ("hobnail") endothelial cells (arrow) surrounded by inflammation
- Clusters of epithelioid endothelial cells may mimic granulomas
- Eosinophils may be prominent

Angiolymphoid hyperplasia with eosinophilia

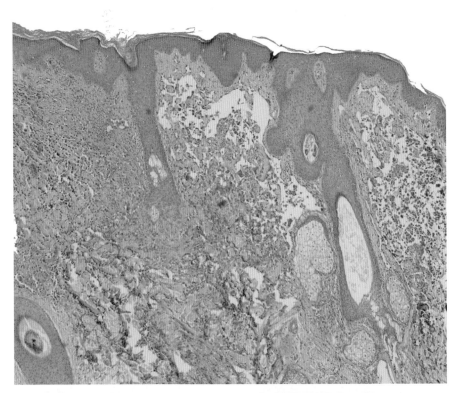

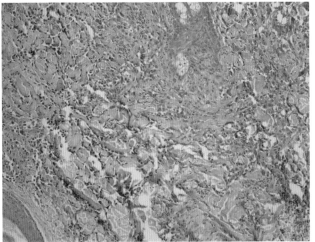

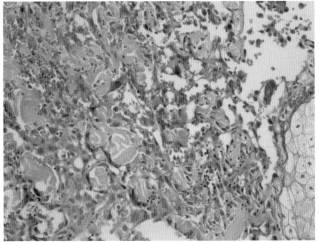

- (Suggestion of) vessels
- Maze-like arrangement of vessels lined by atypical cells
- Deeply infiltrative

Angiosarcoma

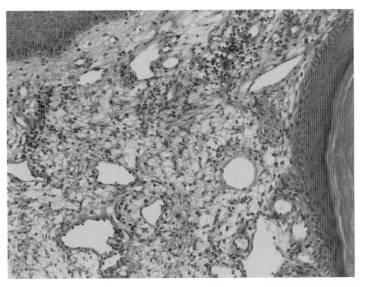

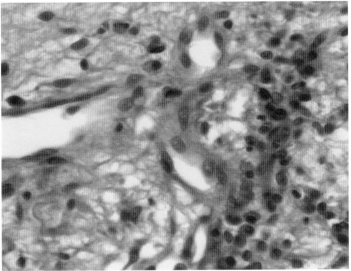

- (Suggestion of) vessels
- Superficial vessels surrounded by plasma cells and red–blue "clouds"/*granular material* of organisms that stain with silver   *⊕ neuts.*

Bacillary angiomatosis

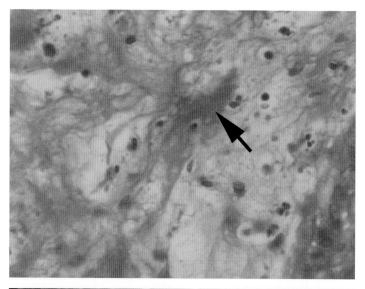

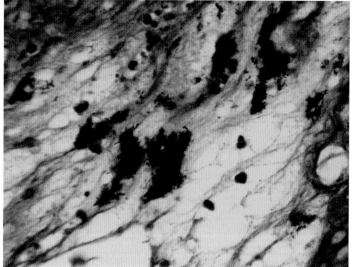

- (Suggestion of) vessels
- Superficial vessels surrounded by plasma cells and red–blue "clouds" of organisms that stain with silver

Bacillary angiomatosis (cont.)

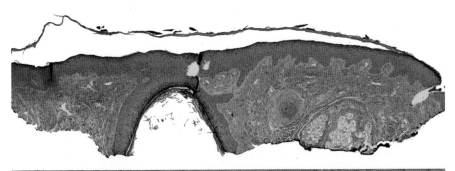

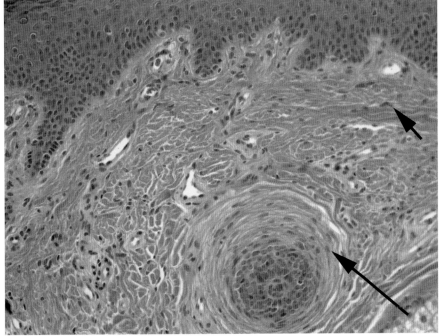

- (Suggestion of) vessels
- Fibrotic stroma
- Concentric fibrosis around vessels/adnexae (long arrow)
- Stellate fibroblasts (short arrow)

Fibrous papule

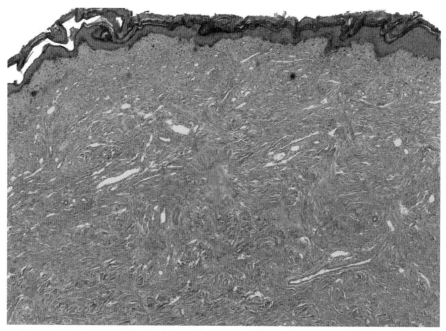

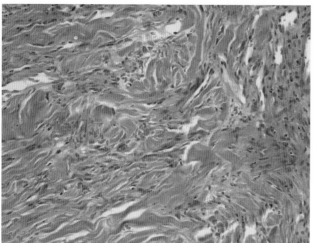
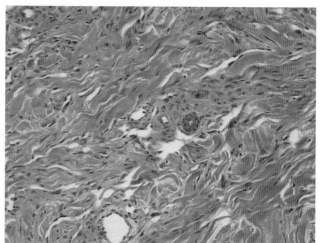

- (Suggestion of) vessels
- Vessels forming around other vessels (promontory sign)
- Vessels may be lined by inconspicuous endothelial cells

Kaposi's sarcoma

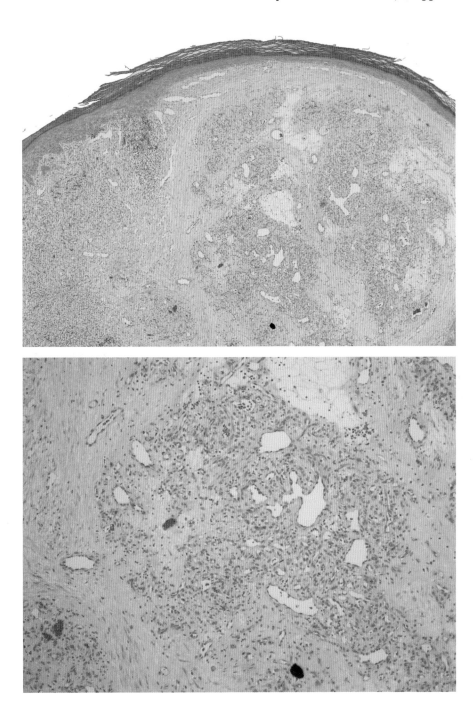

- (Suggestion of) vessels
- Lobules of dilated vessels embedded in loose stroma with inflammatory cells

Pyogenic granuloma

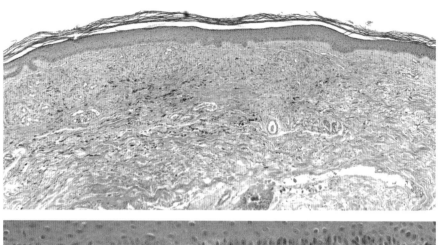

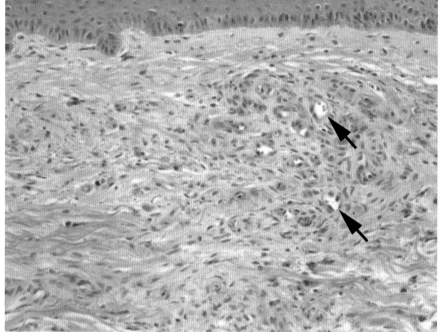

- (Suggestion of) vessels
- Hyperkeratosis
- Variable spongiosis
- Small-caliber thick-walled capillaries in clusters in the upper dermis (arrows)
- Hemosiderin

Stasis dermatitis

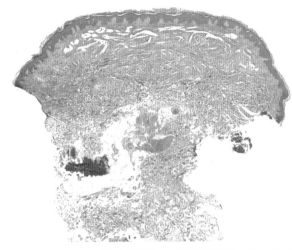

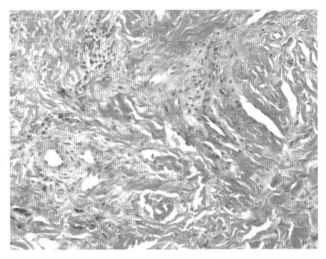

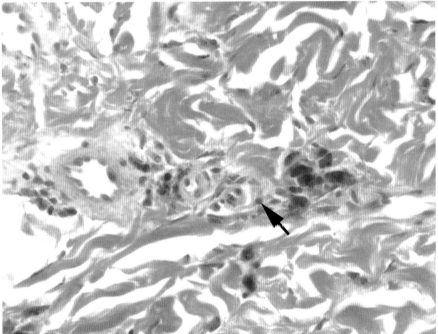

- (Suggestion of) vessels
- Somewhat wedge-shaped arrangement of vessels
- Hemosiderin (arrow) around the peripheral vessels

Targetoid hemangioma

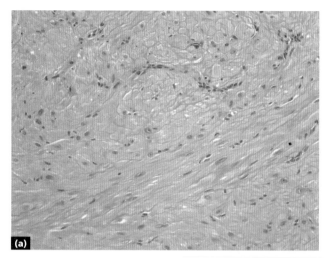

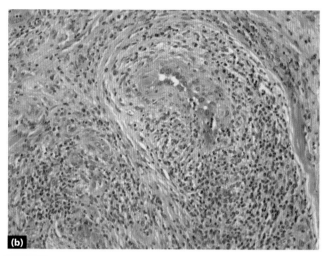

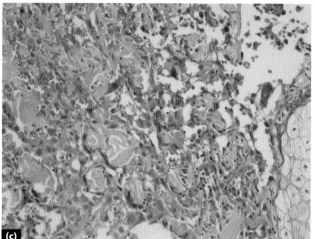

(Suggestion of) vessels

- **a** Angioleiomyoma: well-circumscribed pink circle composed of cigar-shaped spindle cells and compressed to dilated vessels

- **b** Angiolymphoid hyperplasia with eosinophilia: dilated vessels with prominent hobnail endothelial cells surrounded by inflammation, +/− numerous eosinophils
- **c** Angiosarcoma: maze-like connection of vessels lined by atypical cells

Key differences

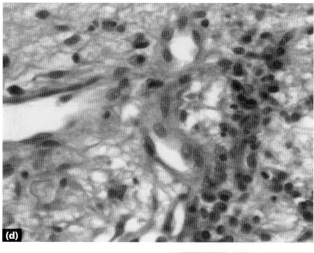

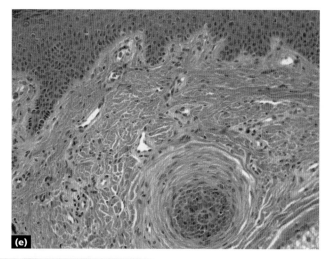

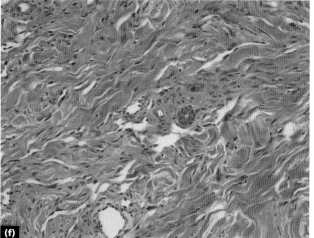

(Suggestion of) vessels (cont.)

- **d** Bacillary angiomatosis: dilated vessels surrounded by inflammation that includes plasma cells and ill-defined "clouds"
- **e** Fibrous papule: fibrotic stroma with stellate fibroblasts and dilated vessels

- **f** Kaposi's sarcoma: slit-like or angulated spaces dissecting through collagen; vessels around vessels

Key differences

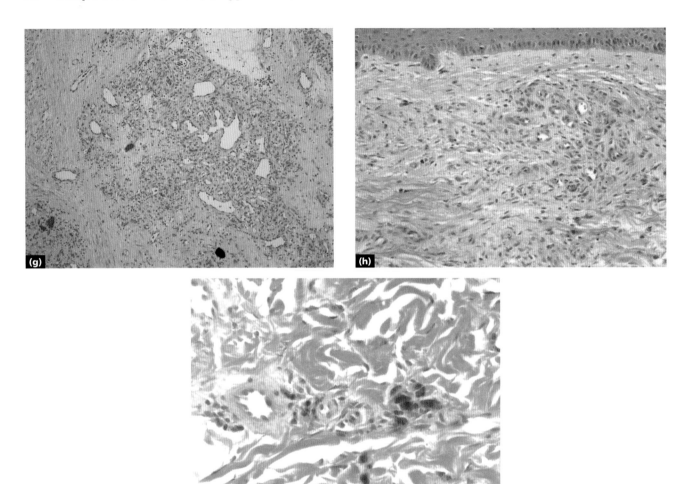

(Suggestion of) vessels (cont.)

- **g** Pyogenic granuloma: clusters of dilated vessels surrounded by mixed inflammation
- **h** Stasis dermatitis: small clusters of capillaries in upper dermis with hemosiderin
- **i** Targetoid hemangioma: wedge-shaped area of increased vessels with hemosiderin at periphery

Key differences

2

Top–Down

- Hyperkeratosis, 85

- Parakeratosis, 94

- Upper epidermal changes, 97

- Acantholysis, 107

- Eosinophilic spongiosis, 117

- Subepidermal space/cleft, 124

- Perivascular infiltrate, 132

- Band-like upper dermal infiltrate, 137

- Interface reaction, 141

- Dermal material, 149

- Change in fat, 162

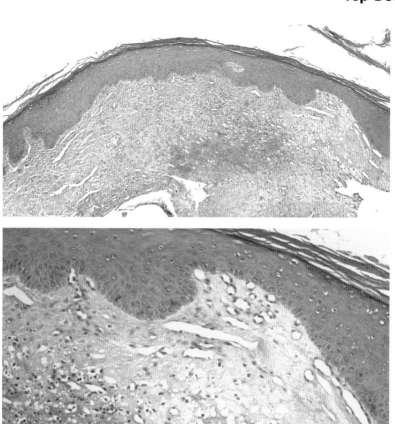

- Hyperkeratosis
- Central erosion/ulceration of epidermis with underlying pink fibrin and flanking vessels
- Vascular ectasia with plump endothelial cells
- Cartilage may be present beneath fibrin

Chondrodermatitis nodularis helicis

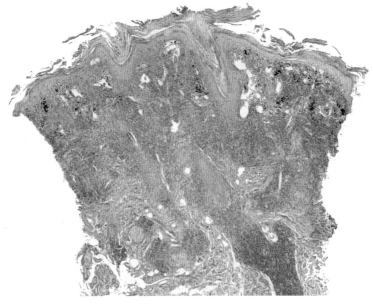

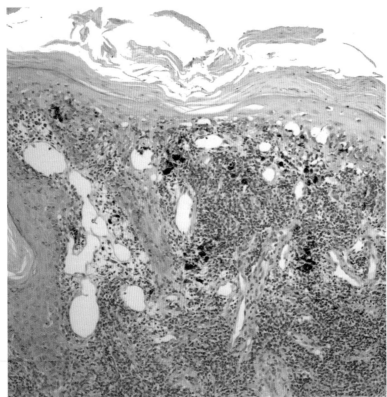

- Hyperkeratosis
- Follicular plugging
- Thinned epidermis
- Vacuolar change at dermoepidermal junction

- Thickened basement membrane
- Pigment incontinence
- Periadnexal and perivascular lymphocytic infiltrate

Discoid lupus erythematosus

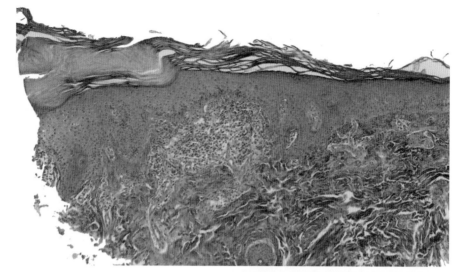

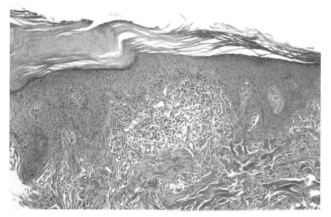
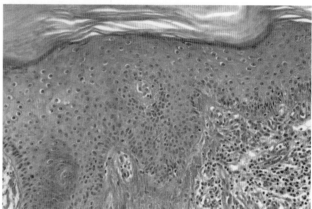

- Hyperkeratosis
- Scattered "dyskeratotic" keratinocytes
- Slightly acanthotic epidermis
- Variable inflammatory infiltrate

Flegel's disease

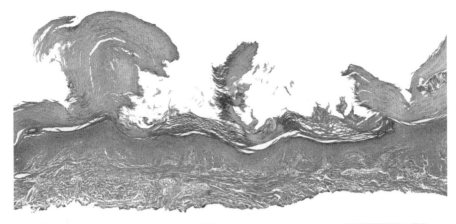

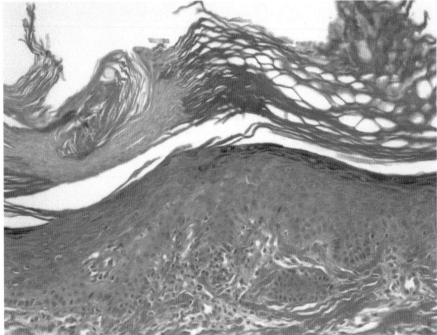

- Hyperkeratosis
- Hyperkeratosis alternates with parakeratosis
- Acanthotic epidermis

Inflammatory linear verrucous epidermal nevus

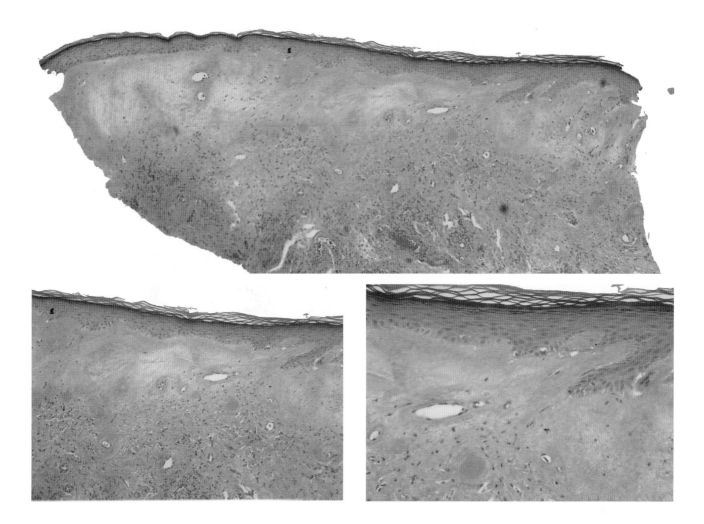

- Hyperkeratosis
- Vacuolar change at dermoepidermal junction
- Pink homogenization of papillary dermis
- Underlying band-like inflammatory infiltrate
- See also p. 264

Lichen sclerosus et atrophicus

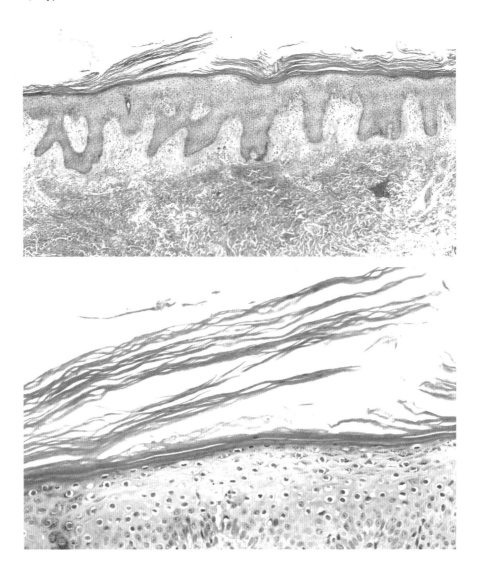

- Hyperkeratosis
- Hyperkeratosis alternates with parakeratosis in a checkerboard pattern
- Follicular plugging
- Irregular acanthosis of epidermis

Pityriasis rubra pilaris

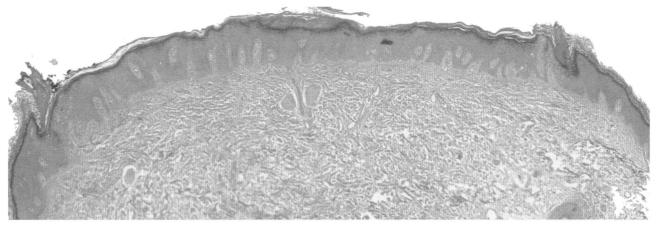

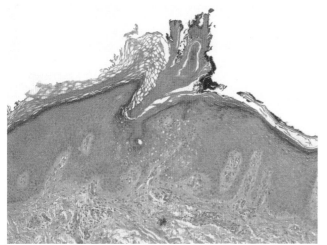
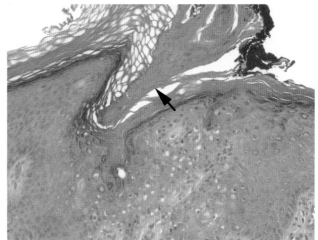

- Hyperkeratosis
- Cornoid lamellae (tiered parakeratosis above altered granular layer) (arrow)
- A lichenoid infiltrate may be present

Porokeratosis

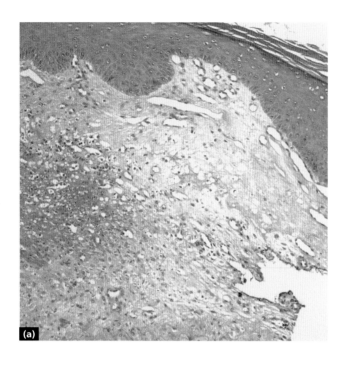

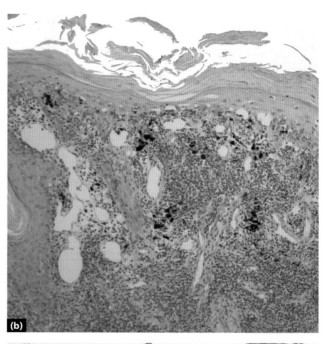

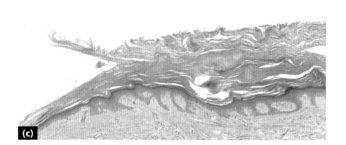

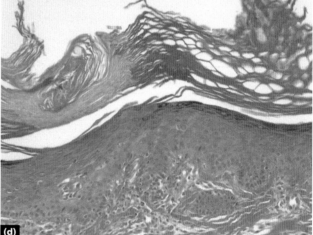

Hyperkeratosis

- **a** Chondrodermatitis nodularis helicis: epidermal erosion/ulceration with underlying fibrin and flanking vessels
- **b** Discoid lupus erythematosus: follicular plugging, thickened basement membrane, periadnexal inflammation
- **c** Flegel's disease: hyperkeratosis over slight acanthosis, minimal inflammation
- **d** Inflammatory linear verrucous epidermal nevus: hyperkeratosis alternating with parakeratosis over acanthosis

Key differences

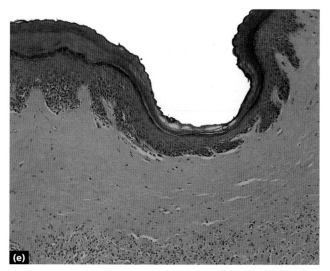

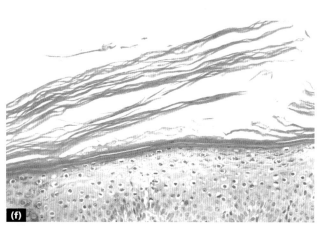

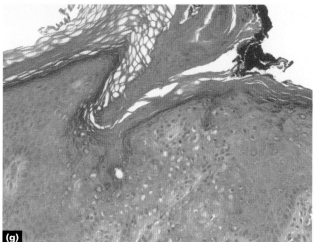

Hyperkeratosis (cont.)

- **e** Lichen sclerosus et atrophicus: pink homogenized papillary dermis with underlying inflammation (see also p. 266)
- **f** Pityriasis rubra pilaris: checkerboard parakeratosis and hyperkeratosis, irregular acanthosis
- **g** Porokeratosis: cornoid lamellae

Key differences

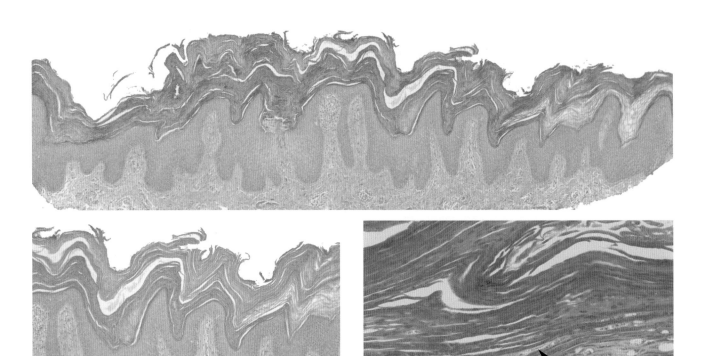

• Parakeratosis
• Granules retained in the stratum corneum (arrows)

Axillary granular parakeratosis

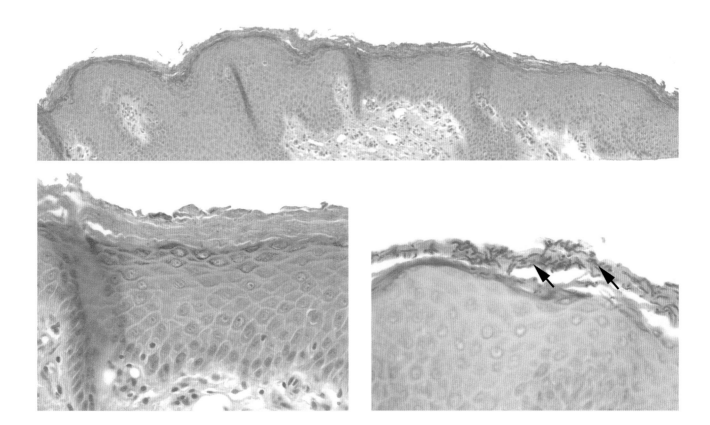

- Parakeratosis may be seen above orthokeratosis ("sandwich sign")
- Slightly refractile organisms (spheres and tubules) in stratum corneum
- Obvious organisms on periodic acid–Schiff (arrows)

Dermatophytosis

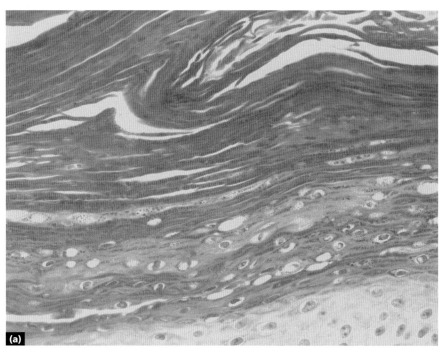

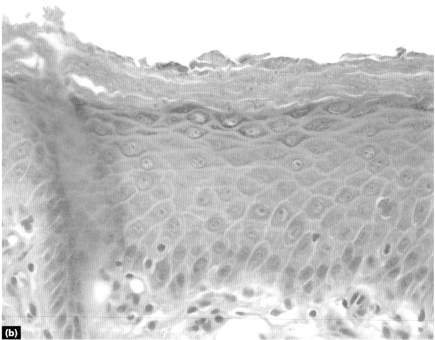

Parakeratosis

- **a** Axillary granular parakeratosis: retained granules in stratum corneum
- **b** Dermatophytosis: circles and linear hyphae in stratum corneum

- **Note** Tinea versicolor is in the differential; dermatophytosis and tinea versicolor may be subtle and appear like "normal" skin on low power

Key differences

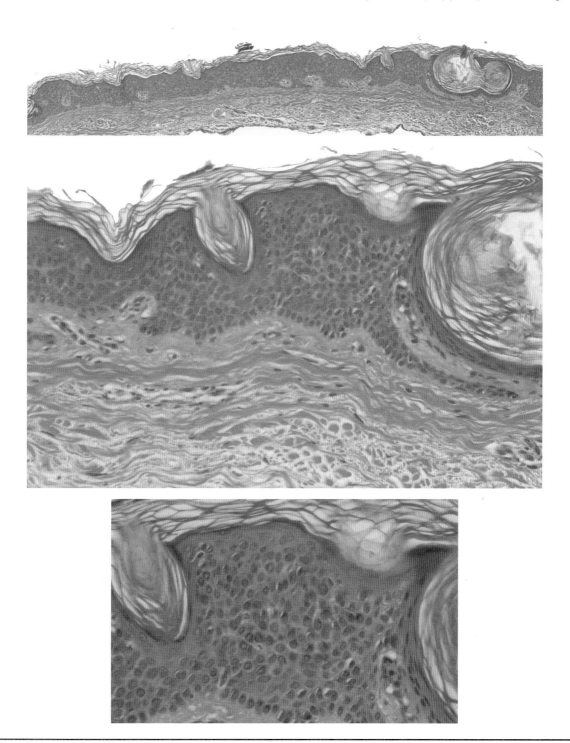

- Upper epidermal change of nests of keratinocytes
- Nests are composed of monomorphous, typical keratinocytes

Clonal seborrheic keratosis

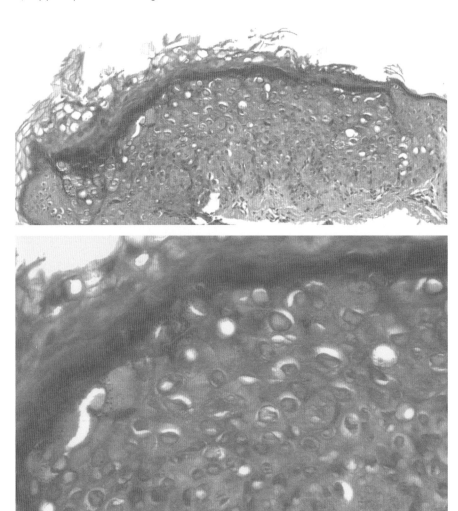

• Upper epidermal change of keratinocytes with blue–gray
  expanded cytoplasm and haloes around nuclei

Epidermodysplasia verruciformis

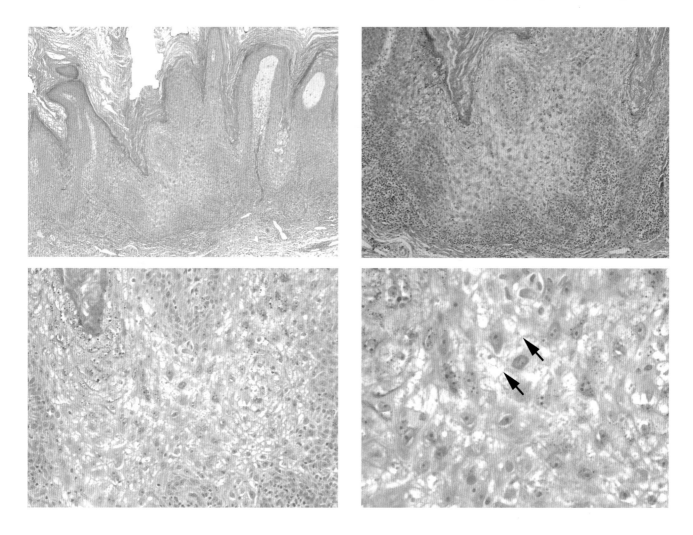

- Upper epidermal change of prominent keratohyaline
  granules and chicken-wire cell membranes –
  granular-vacuolar change (arrows)

Epidermolytic hyperkeratosis

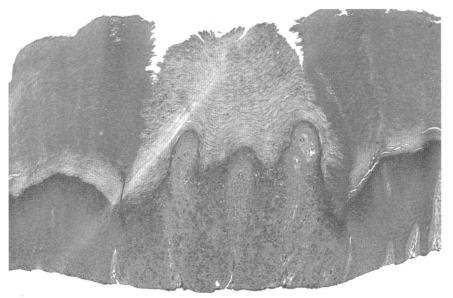

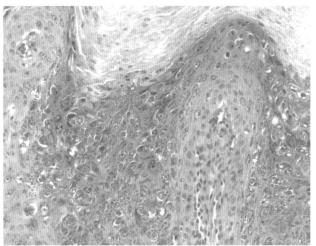
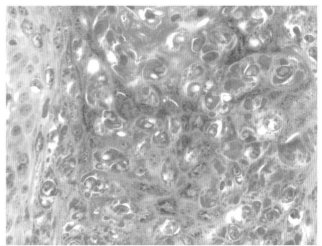

- Upper epidermal change of koilocytes with very prominent keratohyaline granules
- A type of wart that tends to be on the plantar surface

Myrmecium

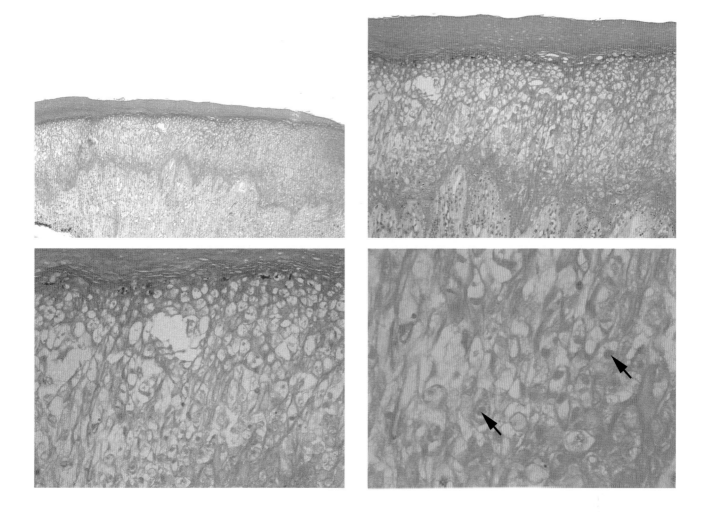

- Upper epidermal change of reticular degeneration
  (edema of the cells with retention of cell membranes) and
  pink intracytoplasmic globules (arrows)
- Usually acral skin

Orf

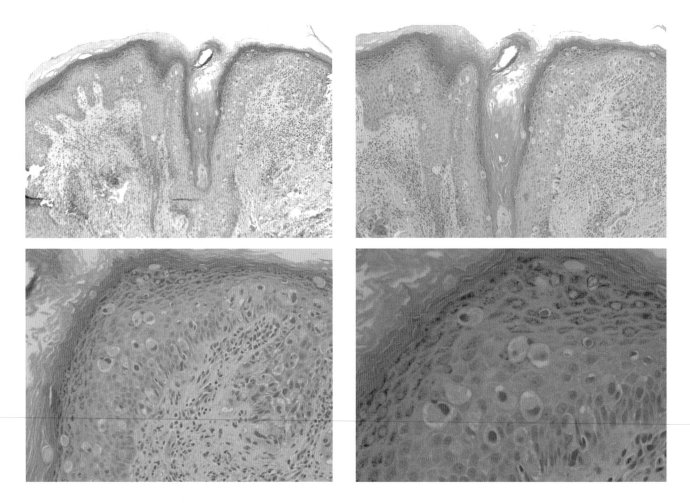

- Upper epidermal change of scattered large cells singly and in nests
- May be able to see a compressed basal layer beneath nests (eye-liner)
- Large cells have expanded cytoplasm and nuclei at periphery

Paget's disease

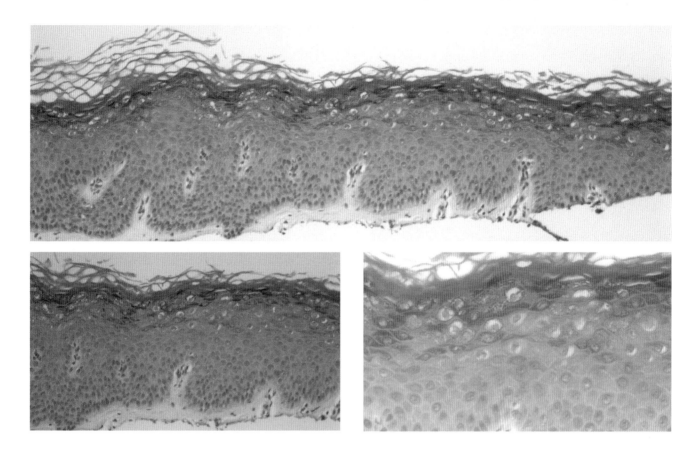

- Upper epidermal change of koilocytes – cells with haloes around nuclei
- Epidermal surface is only slightly papillated

Verruca plana

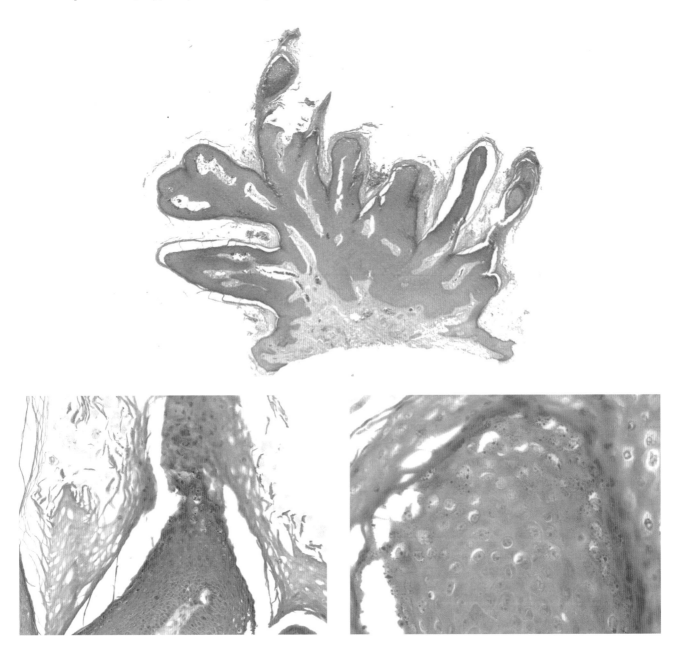

- Upper epidermal change of koilocytes
- Epidermal surface papillated
- Toeing-in (arborization) of rete ridges

Verruca vulgaris

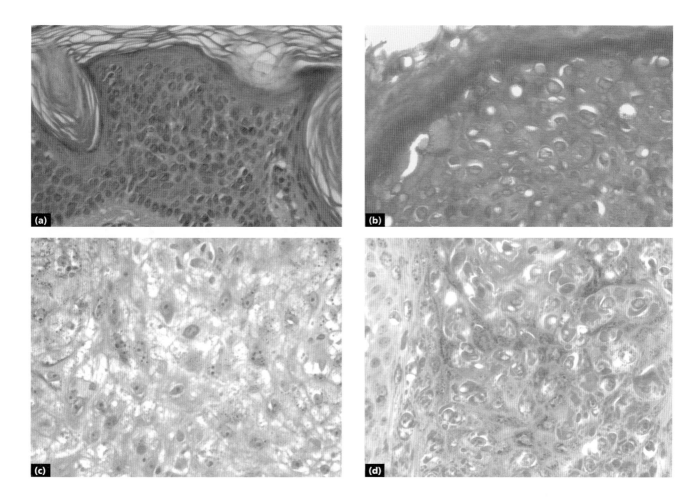

Upper epidermal change

- **a** Clonal seborrheic keratosis: nests of typical, monomorphous keratinocytes
- **b** Epidermodysplasia verruciformis: expanded blue–gray cytoplasm, some perinuclear haloes
- **c** Epidermolytic hyperkeratosis: strung-out cell membranes, loss of nuclei, granular–vacuolar change
- **d** Myrmecium: very prominent keratohyaline granules

Key differences

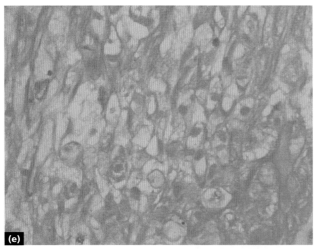

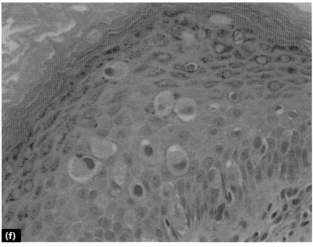

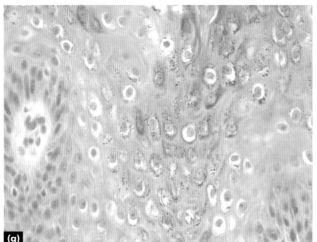

Upper epidermal change (cont.)

- **e** Orf: reticular degeneration (pink cell membranes with loss of nuclei) with scattered inclusions
- **f** Paget's disease: scattered cells that lack intercellular bridges with prominent grayish cytoplasm
- **g** Verruca: koilocytes

Key differences

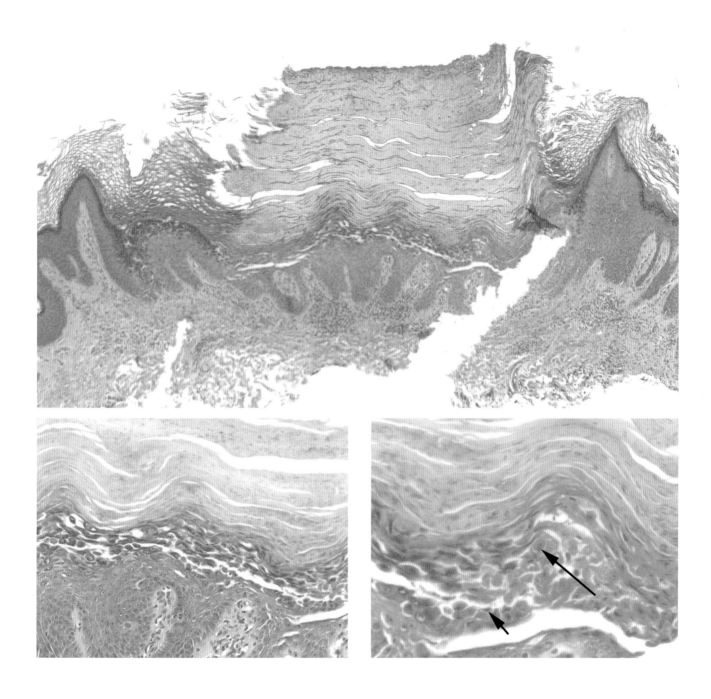

- Benign acantholytic dyskeratosis with corp ronds
  (long arrow) and grains (short arrow)
- Parakeratosis above the acantholytic dyskeratosis

Darier's disease

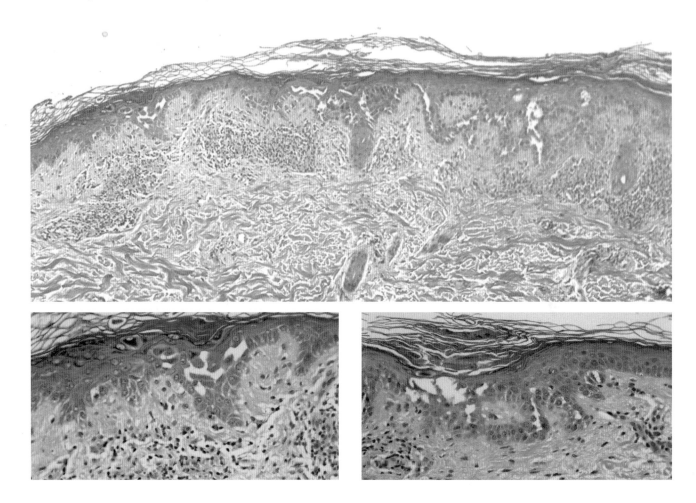

- Benign acantholytic dyskeratosis in small foci
- Also foci of spongiosis, acantholysis without dyskeratosis
  (Hailey–Hailey pattern and pemphigus patterns)

Grover's disease

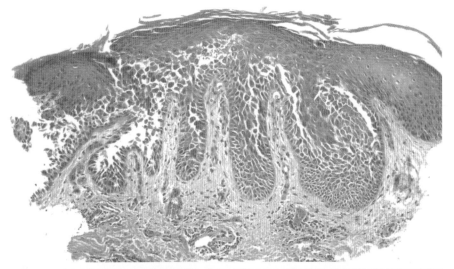

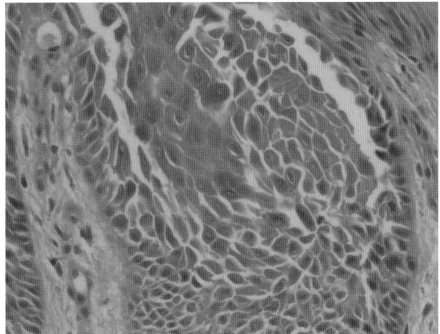

- Benign acantholysis (sometimes with dyskeratosis) in full thickness to two-thirds of the epidermis
- Resembles a "dilapidated brick wall"

Hailey–Hailey disease

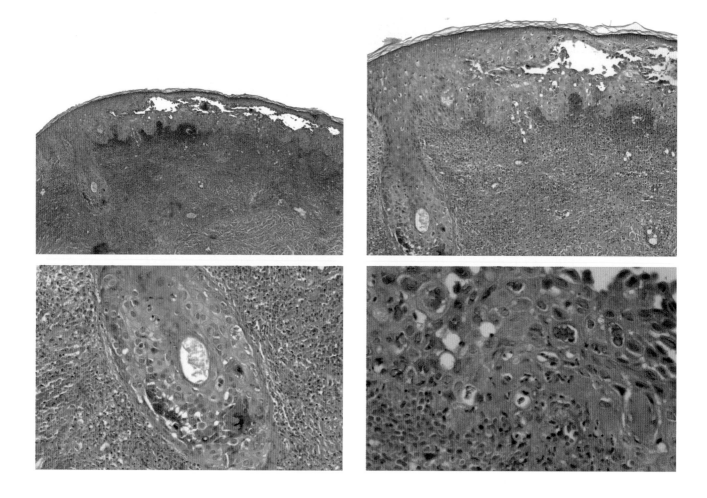

- Benign non-dyskeratotic acantholysis with ballooning
  degeneration
- Multinucleated cells with rimming of chromatin
- Follicular necrosis/acantholysis is a clue

Herpes virus infection

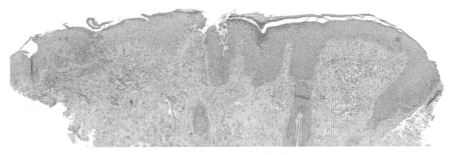

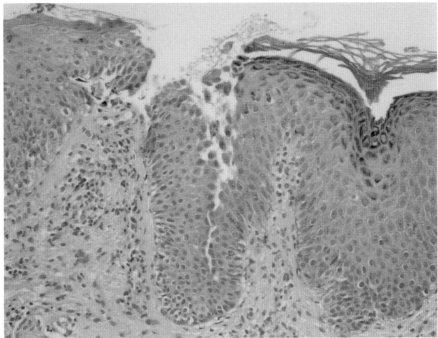

- Benign acantholysis in the upper stratum spinosum, making the granular layer appear altered
- May see "cling-ons" (acantholytic cells on roof of split)

Pemphigus foliaceus

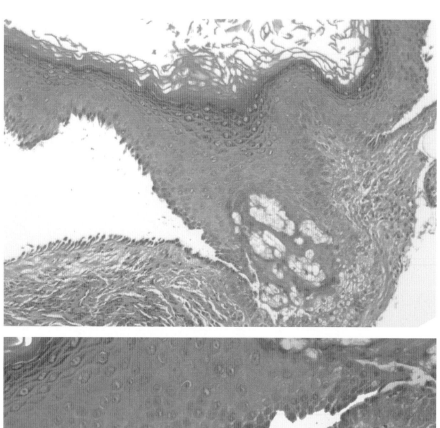

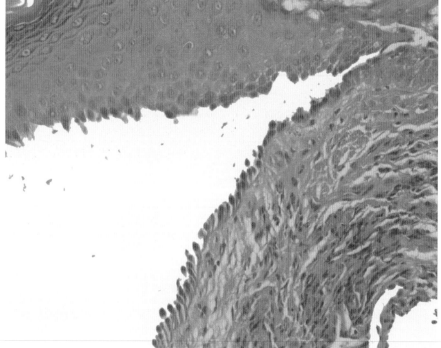

- Benign acantholysis above the basal layer
- Basal layer intact and appears like "tombstones"

Pemphigus vulgaris

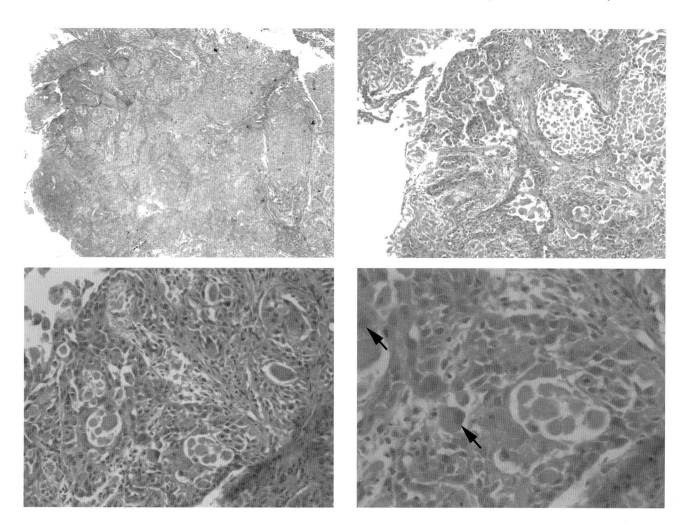

- Malignant dyskeratotic acantholysis in a large, infiltrative tumor
- Prominent atypical cells and mitoses

Squamous cell carcinoma, adenoid type

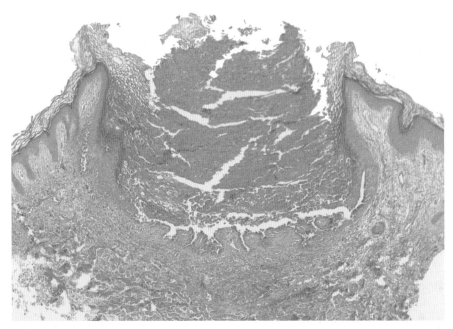

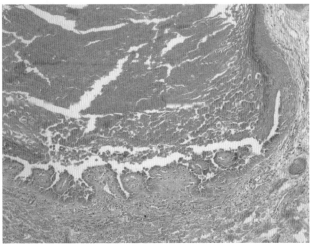

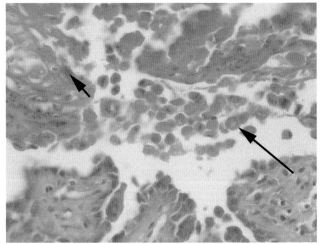

- Benign dyskeratotic acantholysis like Darier's disease with corp ronds (long arrow) and grains (short arrow) but may have more prominent cup-shape and/or follicular involvement
- Clinically a solitary lesion

Warty dyskeratoma

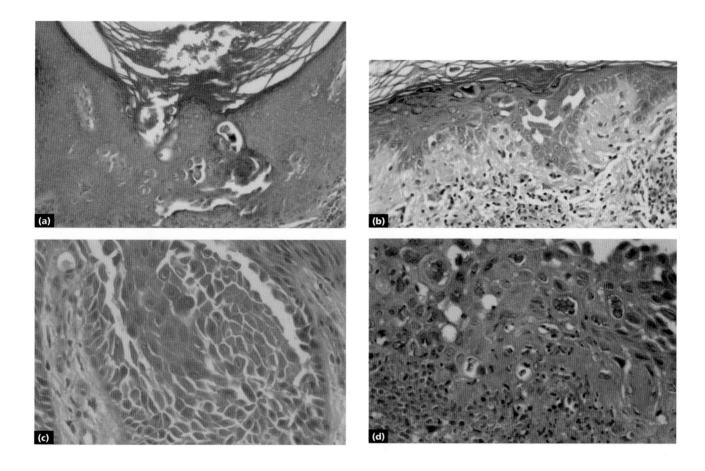

Acantholysis

a Darier's disease: prominent parakeratosis above corp ronds and grains

b Grover's disease: multiple patterns of acantholysis (Darier's-like, Hailey–Hailey-like, pemphigus-like) and spongiosis in small foci

c Hailey–Hailey disease: majority of epidermis involved by acantholysis

d Herpes virus infection: ballooning degeneration, multinucleated cells with chromatin rimming

Key differences

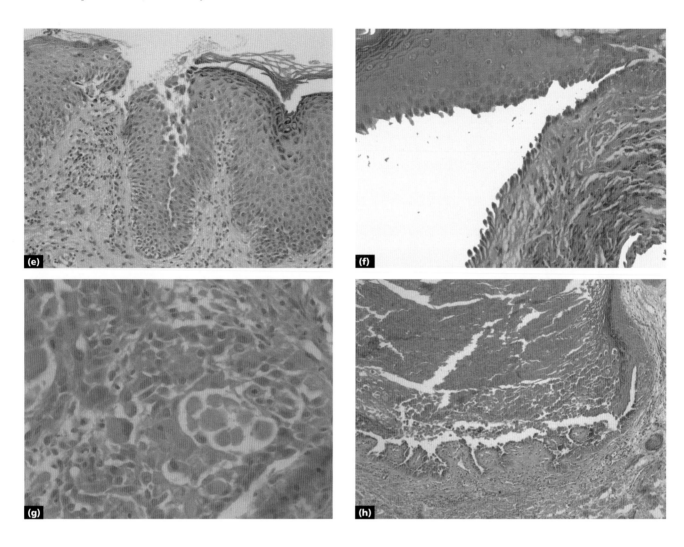

Acantholysis (cont.)

e Pemphigus foliaceus: granular layer prominent with acantholysis

f Pemphigus vulgaris: acantholysis above tombstoned basal layer; follicles may be involved

g Squamous cell carcinoma, adenoid type: acantholysis and squamous pearls, atypical keratinocytes and mitoses (malignant dyskeratotic acantholysis)

h Warty dyskeratoma: cup-shaped area of acantholytic dyskeratosis, villi at base

Key differences

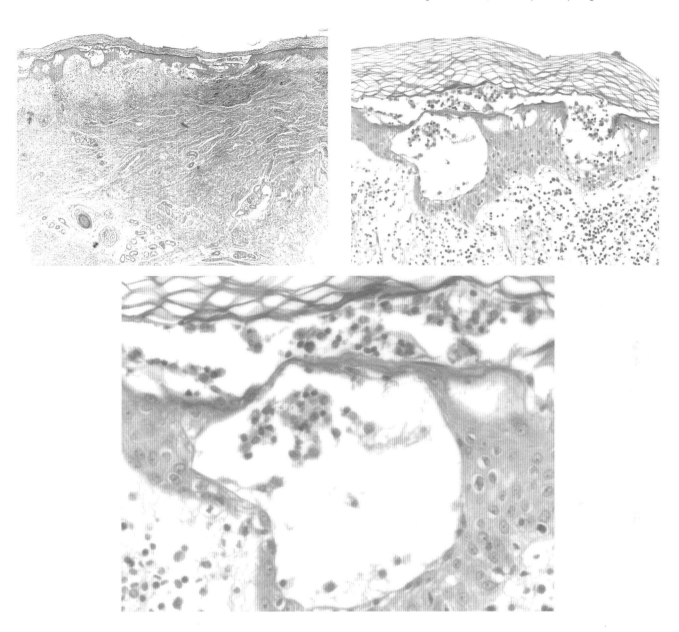

- Eosinophilic spongiosis
- Vesicles within epidermis may be prominent

Allergic contact dermatitis

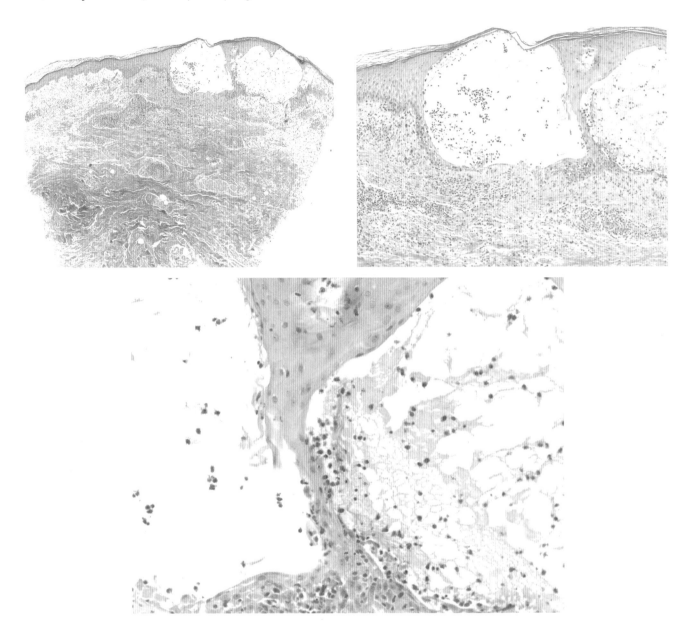

- Eosinophilic spongiosis
- Wedge-shaped pattern of inflammation on low-power view
- Vesicles within epidermis may be prominent

Arthropod bite reaction

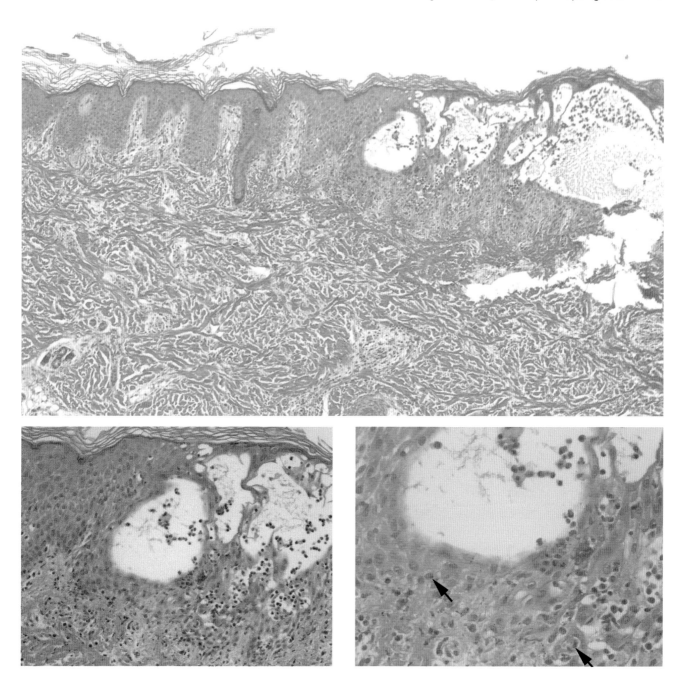

- Eosinophilic spongiosis
- Dyskeratotic keratinocytes (arrows)

Incontinentia pigmenti

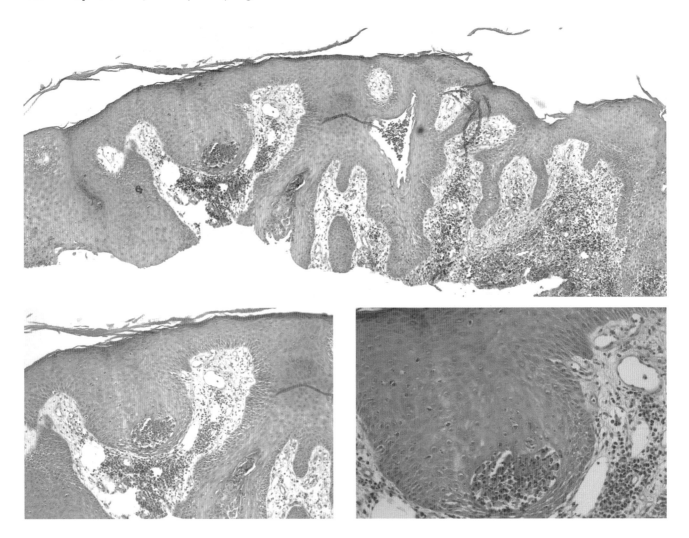

- Eosinophilic abscesses within epidermis
- Acantholysis may be absent to subtle
- Hyperplastic epidermis

Pemphigus vegetans

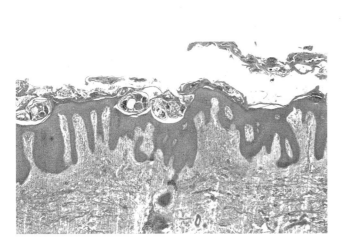
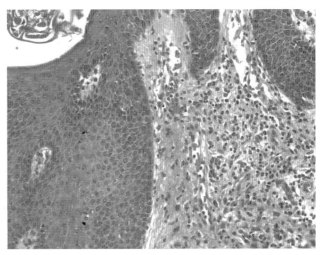
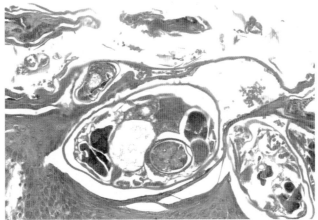

- Eosinophilic spongiosis
- Mites, scybala, eggs within stratum corneum

Scabies

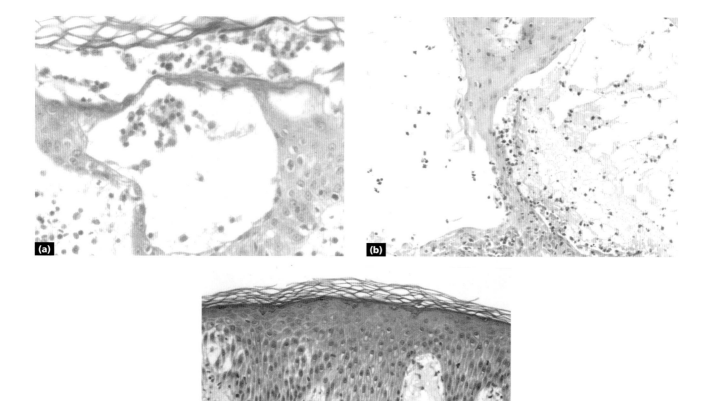

Eosinophilic spongiosis

a Allergic contact dermatitis: orderly vesicles and eosinophils
  in epidermis

b Arthropod bite reaction: prominent vesicles and eosinophils
  in epidermis, may see an erosion

c Bullous pemphigoid: subepidermal cleft and eosinophils
  at base (see also p. 125)

Key differences

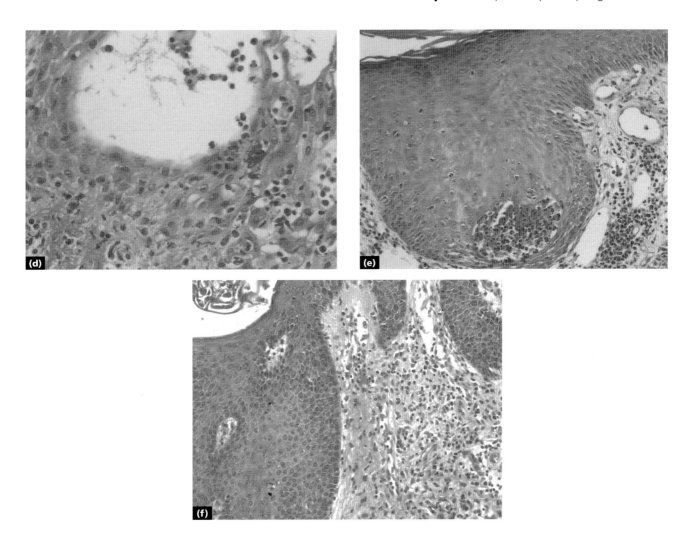

Eosinophilic spongiosis (cont.)

d Incontinentia pigmenti: eosinophilic spongiosis with dyskeratotic cells

e Pemphigus vegetans: eosinophilic abscesses within acanthotic epidermis

f Scabies: mites/scybala/eggs in stratum corneum

Key differences

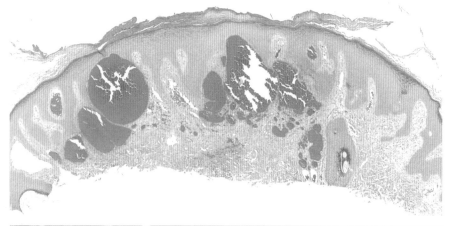

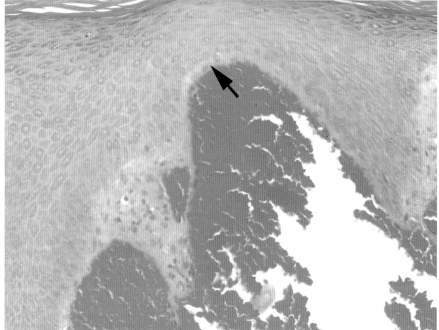

- Subepidermal space (can appear intraepidermal)
- Thin "grenz zone" (arrow)
- Filled with erythrocytes

Angiokeratoma

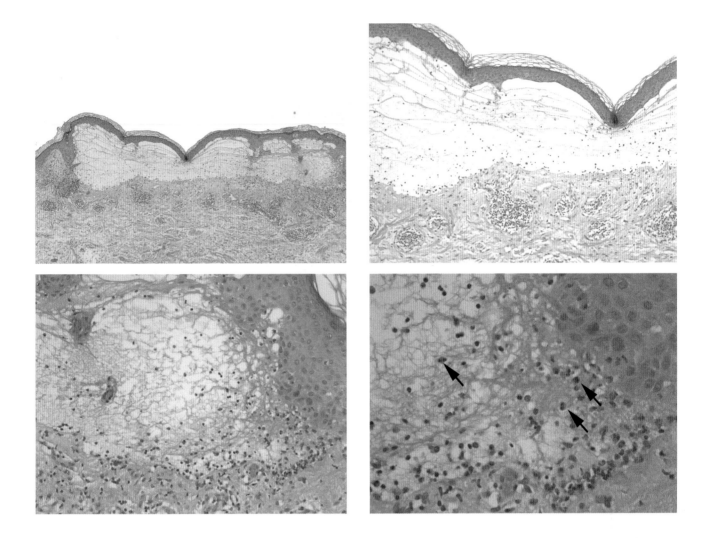

- Subepidermal space
- Eosinophils (arrows) are prominent at the base
- May see festooning (papillated bulla base)

Bullous pemphigoid/Herpes gestationis

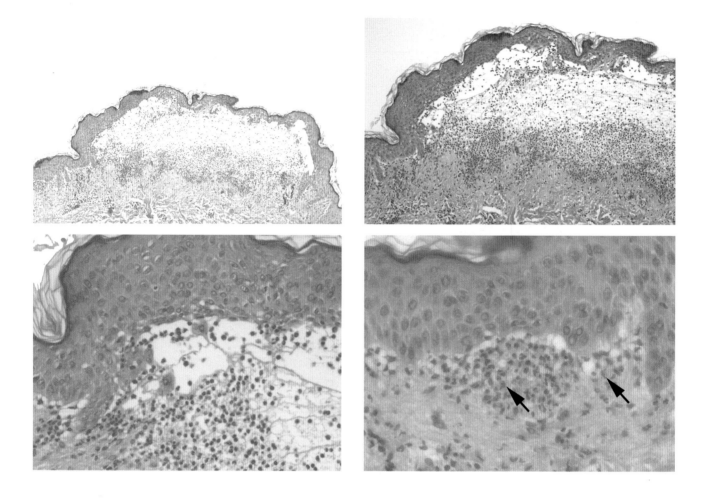

- Subepidermal space
- Neutrophils (arrows) are prominent at the base
- May see clusters of neutrophils in papillae adjacent to blister

- Note that this same histologic pattern can be seen with linear immunoglobulin A disease, neutrophil-rich bullous pemphigoid, bullous lupus erythematosus, and epidermolysis bullosa acquisita
- May see reverse festooning (papillated inferior surface of bulla roof)

Dermatitis herpetiformis

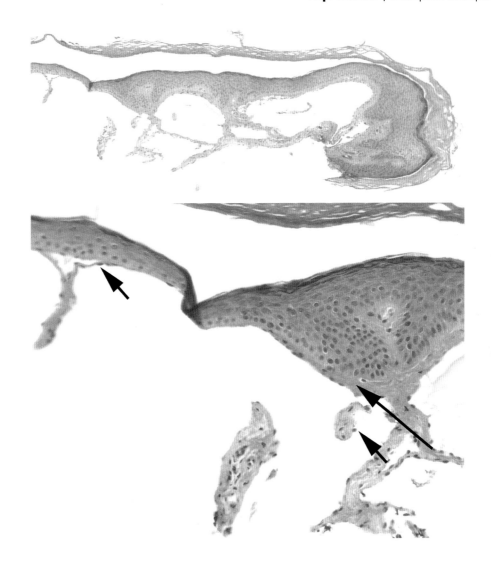

- Subepidermal space with internal papillations
- Thin "grenz zone" (long arrow)
- Spaces lined by endothelial cells (short arrows) and may contain a few erythrocytes

Lymphangioma

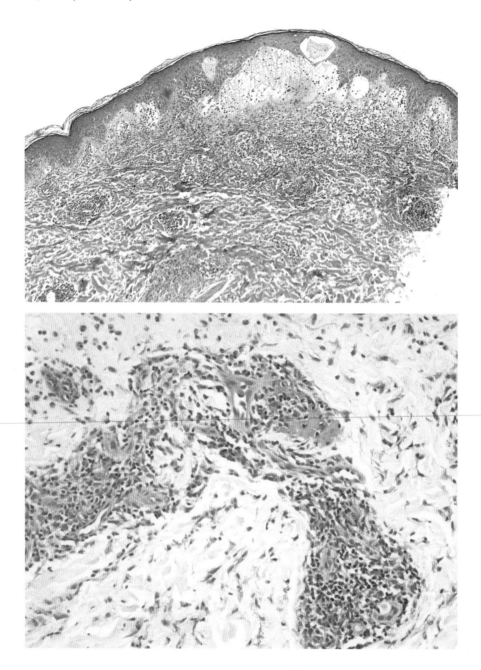

- Subepidermal space (edema)
- Superficial and deep vessels surrounded by lymphocytes

Polymorphous light eruption

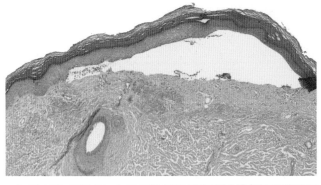

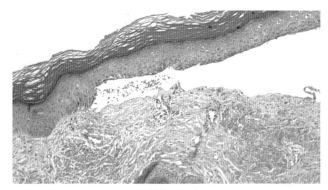

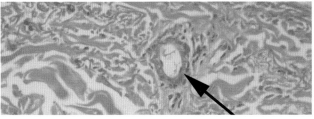

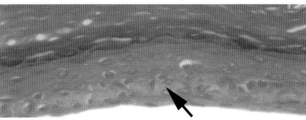

- Subepidermal space
- Often a non-inflammatory base
- Festooning of papillary dermis
- Thickened vessel walls (long arrow)
- Caterpillar bodies in epidermis (short arrow)

- Note that the differential diagnosis of non-inflammatory subepidermal bullae includes non-inflammatory bullous pemphigoid, epidermolysis bullosa acquisita, diabetic bullae, and epidermolysis bullosa subtypes

Porphyria cutanea tarda

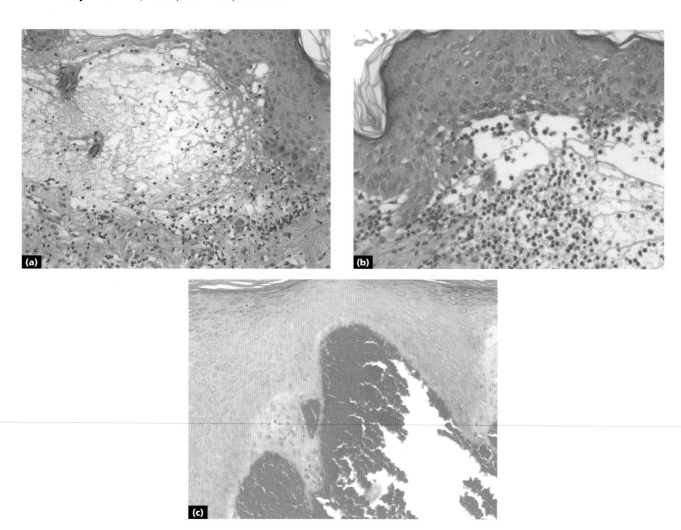

Subepidermal space/cleft

a Bullous pemphigoid: eosinophils at base, festooning
b Dermatitis herpetiformis: neutrophils at base, reverse
  festooning
c Angiokeratoma: erythrocytes fill the spaces

Key differences

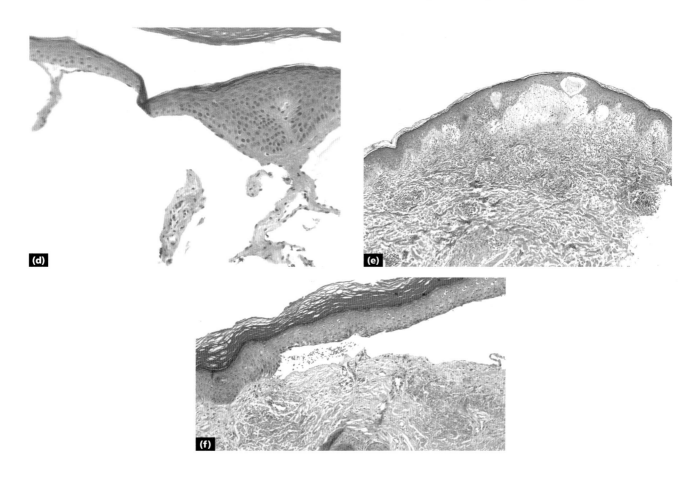

Subepidermal space/cleft (cont.)

d Lymphangioma: spaces lined by endothelial cells and are empty

e Polymorphous light eruption: perivascular lymphocytes

f Porphyria cutanea tarda: non-inflammatory base, festooning, caterpillar bodies

Key differences

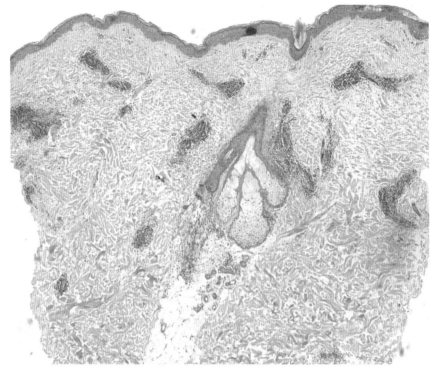

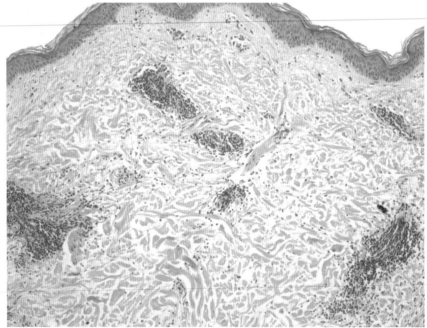

- Superficial and deep perivascular infiltrate of lymphocytes
- Lymphocytes tightly cuffed around vessels
- Note that the differential diagnosis includes polymorphous light eruption (classically has dermal edema), Jessner's lymphocytic infiltrate, and connective tissue disorders

Gyrate erythema

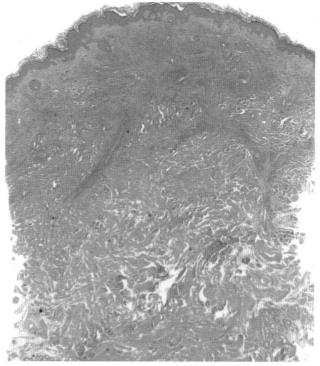

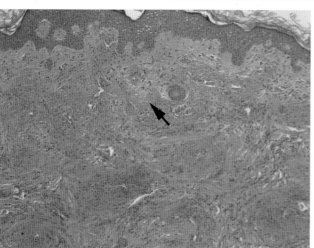

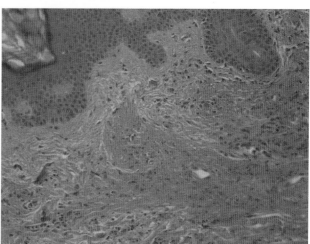

- Perivascular infiltrate of neutrophils and nuclear debris
- Alteration/necrosis of collagen (arrow)
- Extravasated erythrocytes
- Fibrin within vessels

Leukocytoclastic vasculitis

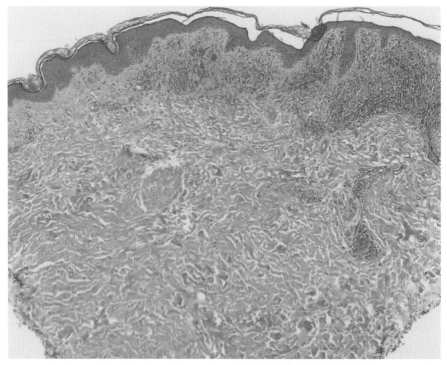

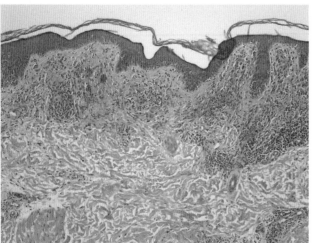

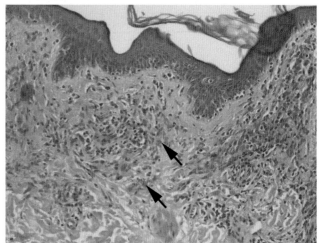

- Superficial perivascular infiltrate of lymphocytes
  (sometimes minimal)
- Extravasated erythrocytes (arrows)
- Hemosiderophages

Pigmented purpuric dermatosis

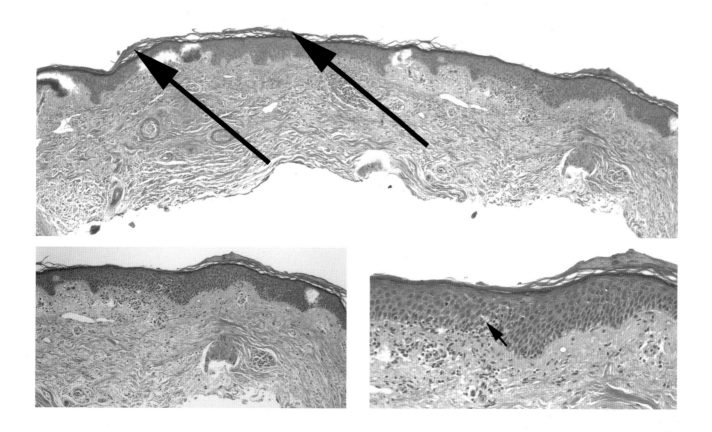

- Superficial perivascular infiltrate of lymphocytes
- Mounds of parakeratosis (long arrows)
- Mild epidermal spongiosis (short arrow)
- Extravasated erythrocytes

- Note that guttate psoriasis is in the differential diagnosis; guttate psoriasis is favored if there are neutrophils in the mounds of parakeratosis

Pityriasis rosea

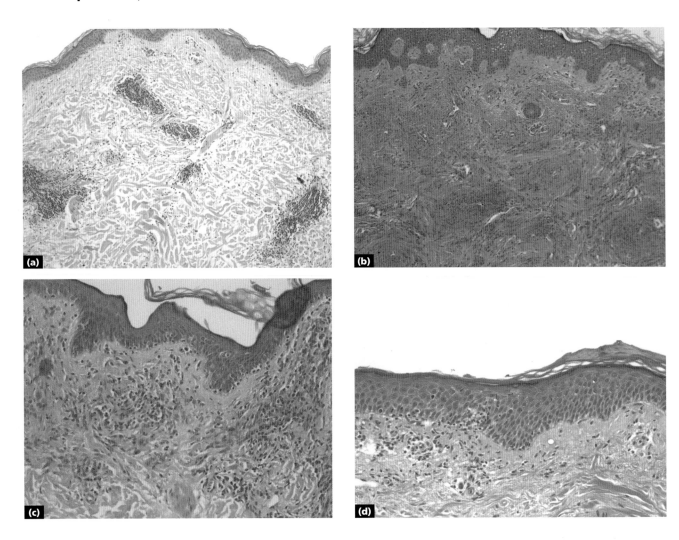

Superficial perivascular infiltrate

- **a** Gyrate erythema: tightly cuffed superficial and deep perivascular infiltrate of lymphocytes, epidermis is normal
- **b** Leukocytoclastic vasculitis: dermis looks "messy" on low power with perivascular neutrophils and nuclear debris, pink donuts of degenerated collagen, extravasated erythrocytes

- **c** Pigmented purpuric dermatosis: perivascular (to lichenoid) infiltrate of lymphocytes, extravasated erythrocytes, hemosiderophages
- **d** Pityriasis rosea: mounds of parakeratosis, mild epidermal spongiosis superficial perivascular infiltrate of lymphocytes, and extravasated erythrocytes
- **Note** Lymphocytic angiitis describes a pattern of perivascular lymphocytes and is a non-diagnostic finding as many diseases may have such a pattern

Key differences

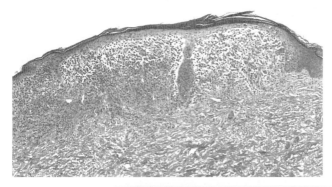
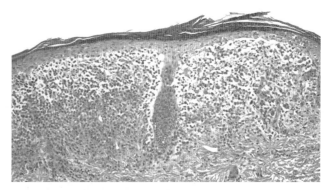
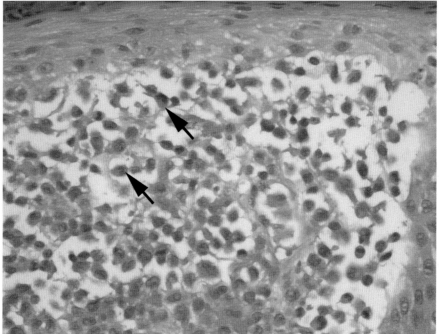

- Band-like upper dermal infiltrate
- Infiltrate abuts and involves epidermis
- Cells in infiltrate have kidney-shaped nuclei (arrows)
- Eosinophils may be present

Langerhans cell histiocytosis

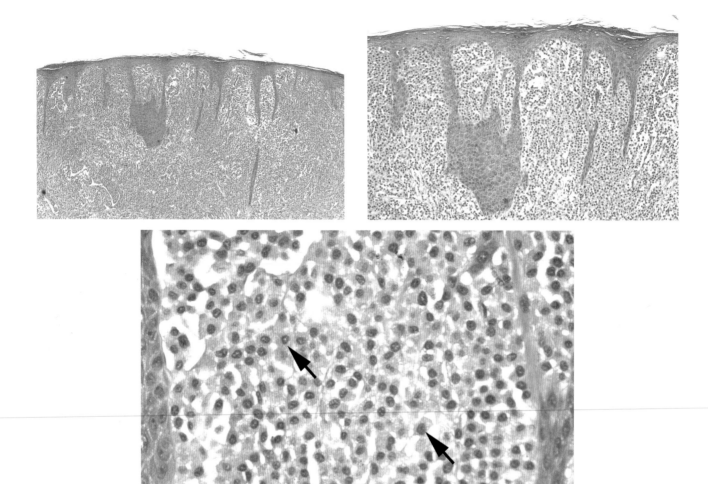

- Band-like upper dermal infiltrate
- A small grenz zone is usually present
- Cells in infiltrate have round nuclei and granular gray–blue cytoplasm (arrows)
- Eosinophils may be present

Mastocytosis

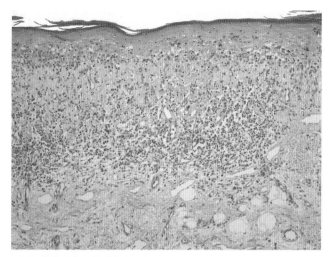

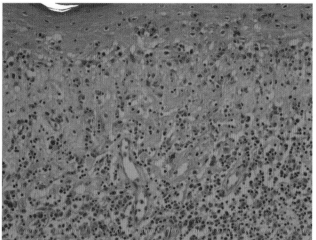

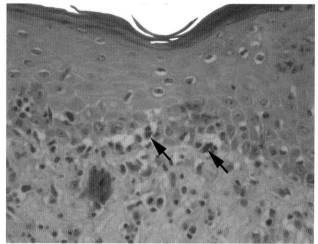

- Band-like upper dermal infiltrate
- Infiltrate abuts and involves epidermis
- May see Pautrier's microabscesses
- Cells in infiltrate have atypical nuclei (arrows)

Mycosis fungoides

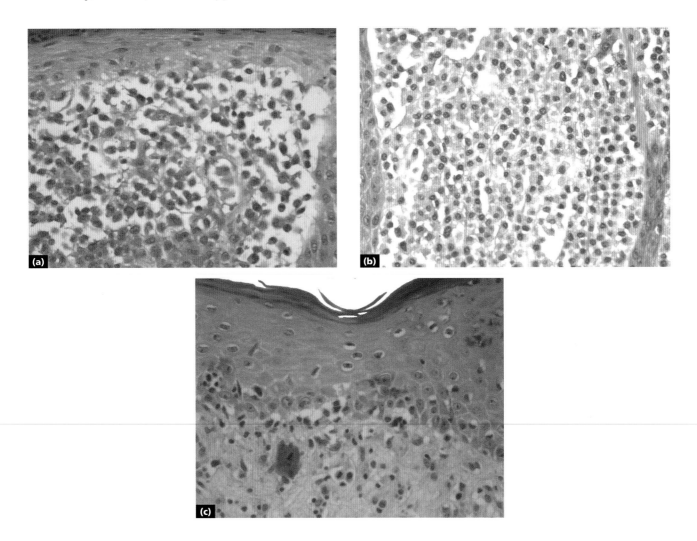

Band-like upper dermal infiltrate
- **a** Langerhans cell histiocytosis: kidney-shaped nuclei
- **b** Mastocytosis: round nuclei and slightly granular cytoplasm
- **c** Mycosis fungoides: cells in infiltrate have atypical nuclei,
  vacuolar change, fibrosis in dermis, lining up of lymphocytes
  at dermoepidermal junction

Key differences

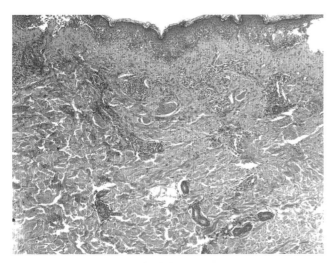
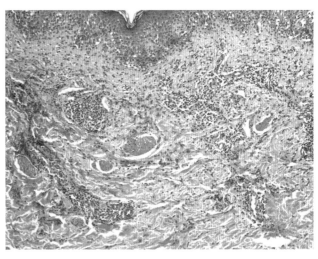
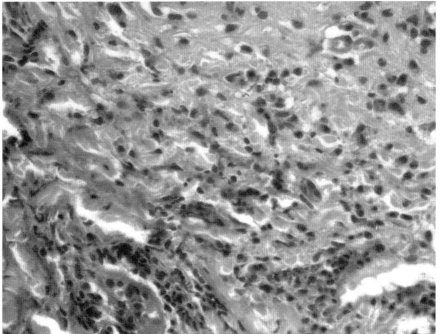

- Interface reaction
- Lichenoid infiltrate
- Numerous necrotic keratinocytes
- Incontinence of pigment
- Deep perivascular infiltrate
- Infiltrate is mixed with eosinophils

Fixed drug reaction

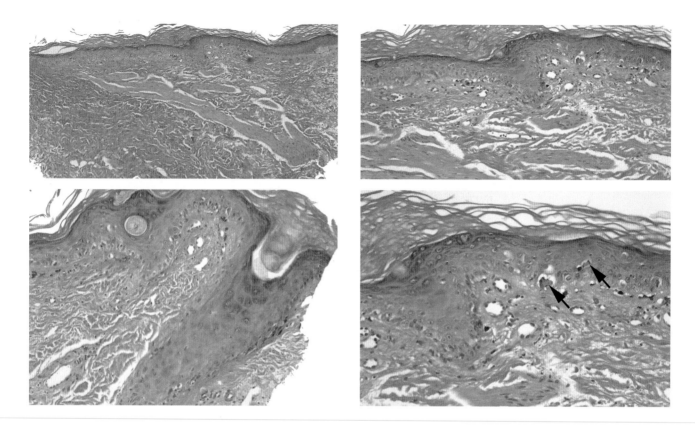

- Interface reaction
- Vacuolar change at dermoepidermal junction
- Necrotic keratinocytes (arrows) in epidermis and follicles
  surrounded by lymphocytes (satellite cell necrosis)

Graft-versus-host disease

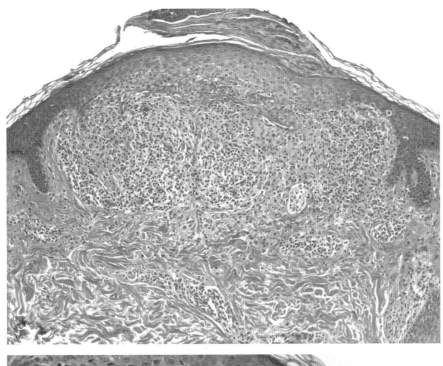

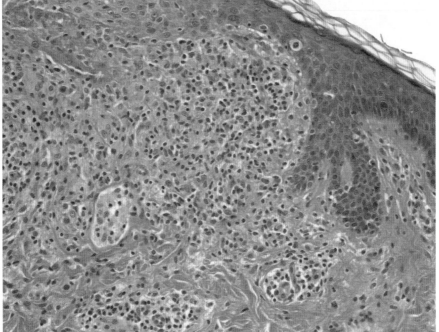

- Interface reaction
- Lichenoid infiltrate that is the "ball" being held by fingers of epidermis (the "claw")
- Infiltrate is composed of lymphocytes and histiocytes and occasional giant cells

Lichen nitidus

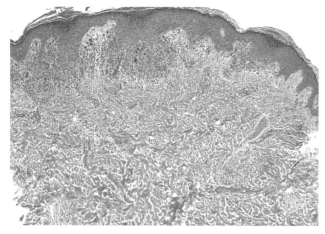

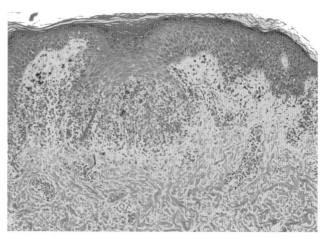

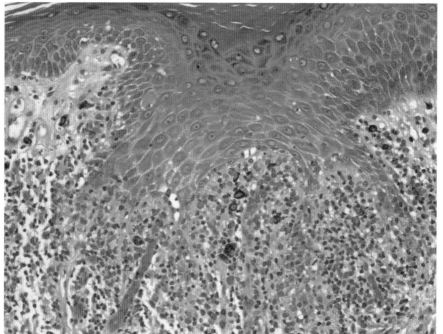

- Interface reaction
- Lichenoid infiltrate
- Hyperkeratosis, irregular acanthosis, hypergranulosis
- Saw-toothing of basal layer
- Colloid bodies, Civatte bodies
- Pigment incontinence

- Usually no eosinophils
- If a mucosal surface, plasma cells may be present
- Note that lichenoid drug reactions can look the same but usually show parakeratosis and eosinophils
- Note that benign lichenoid keratosis can look the same (need clinical history)

Lichen planus

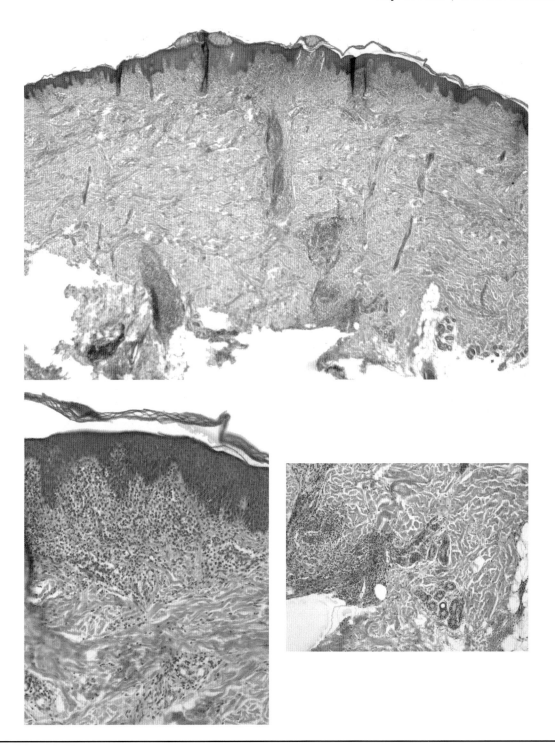

- Interface reaction
- Lichenoid infiltrate and deep perivascular/periadnexal infiltrate
- Peri-eccrine lymphocytic infiltrate is a clue
- Scattered (high and low) apoptotic keratinocytes

Lichen striatus

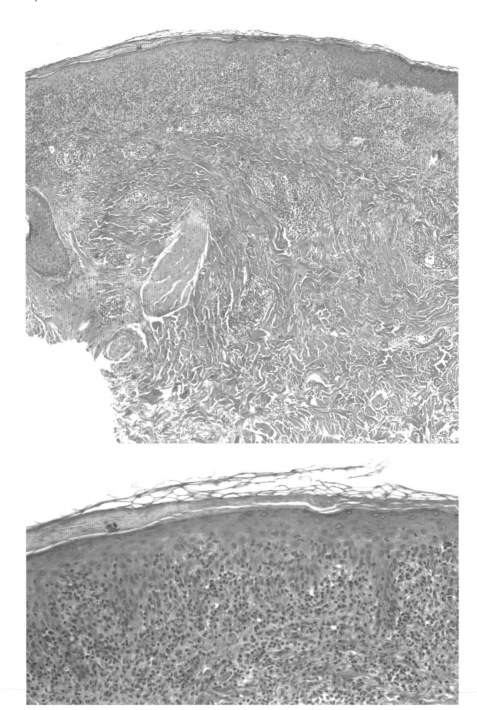

- Interface reaction
- Lichenoid and deep perivascular lymphocytic infiltrate
  (wedge shaped on low power)
- Parakeratosis
- Erythrocytes in the epidermis and extravasated in the dermis
- Necrosis of the epidermis

Pityriasis lichenoides et varioliformis acuta

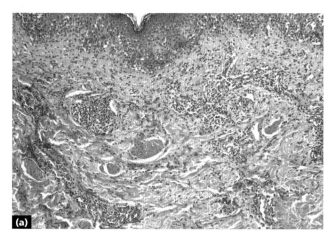

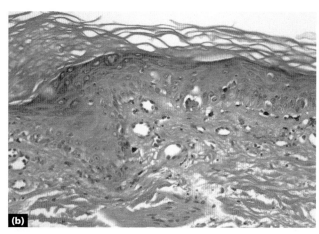

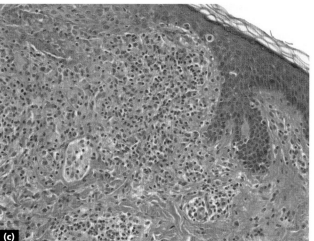

Interface reaction

- **a** Fixed drug reaction: lichenoid and deep perivascular mixed infiltrate with eosinophils, linear necrosis of basal cells
- **b** Graft-versus-host disease: vacuolar change with scattered necrotic keratinocytes in epidermis and hair follicles (satellite cell necrosis)

- **c** Lichen nitidus: ball of lymphocytes and histiocytes in the dermis held by an epidermal claw

Key differences

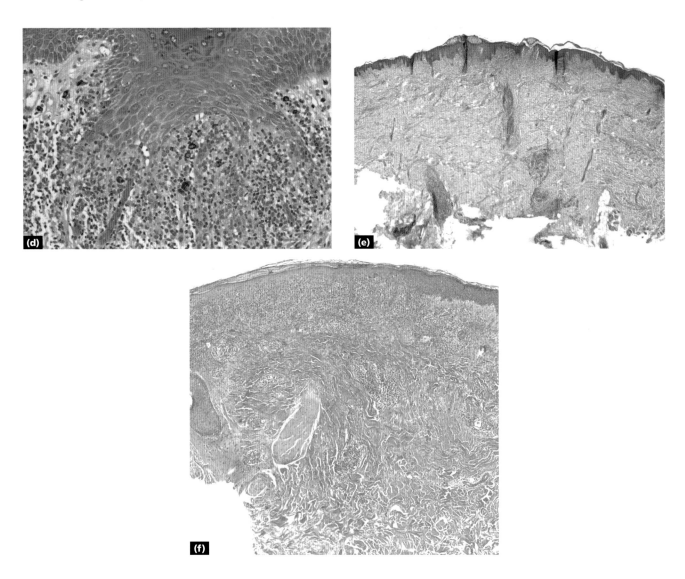

Interface reaction (cont.)

- **d** Lichen planus: lichenoid infiltrate, hyperkeratosis, hypergranulosis, saw-toothed base of acanthotic epidermis
- **e** Lichen striatus: lichenoid and deep infiltrate that involves eccrine glands, scattered necrotic keratinocytes
- **f** Pityriasis lichenoides et varioliformis acuta: parakeratosis, necrotic epidermis, extravasated erythrocytes, lichenoid and deep lymphocytic infiltrate
- **Note** Apoptosis is the type of keratinocyte necrosis seen in interface dermatitis

Key differences

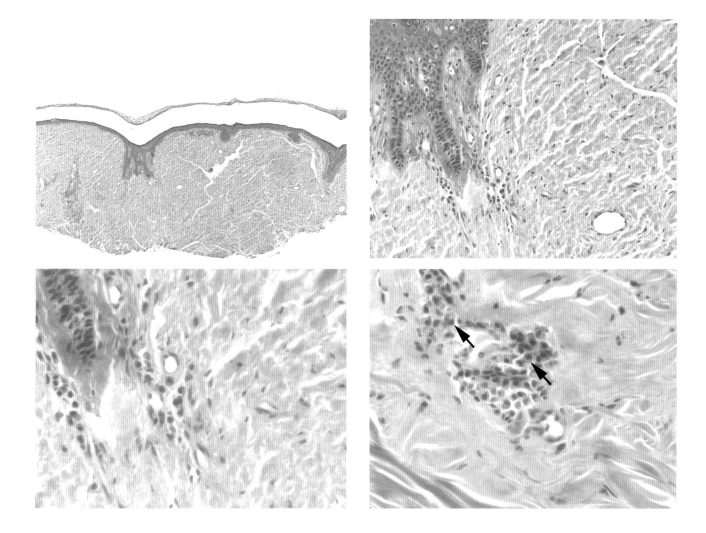

- Dermal material that is pink and amorphous, diffuse, and perivascular
- Plasma cells (arrows) are often present around vessels

Amyloidosis, nodular

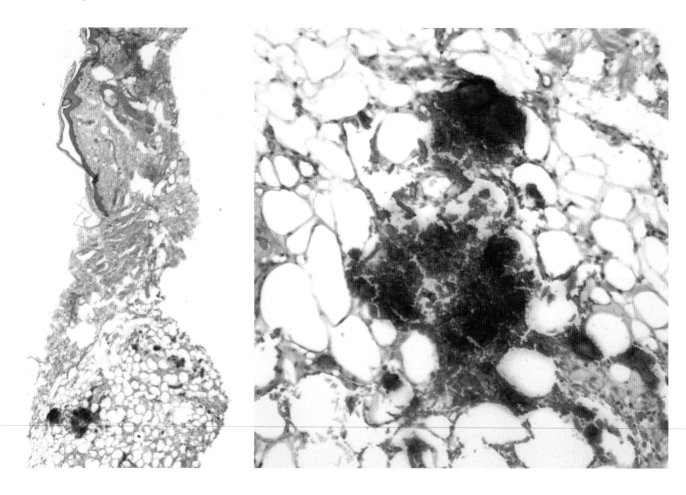

- Dermal material that is blue–purple and chunky
- Calcium deposits can be seen in adnexal tumors (trichoepithelioma, pilomatrixoma)
- Calcium may be deposited on the altered elastic fibers in pseudoxanthoma elasticum

Calcinosis cutis

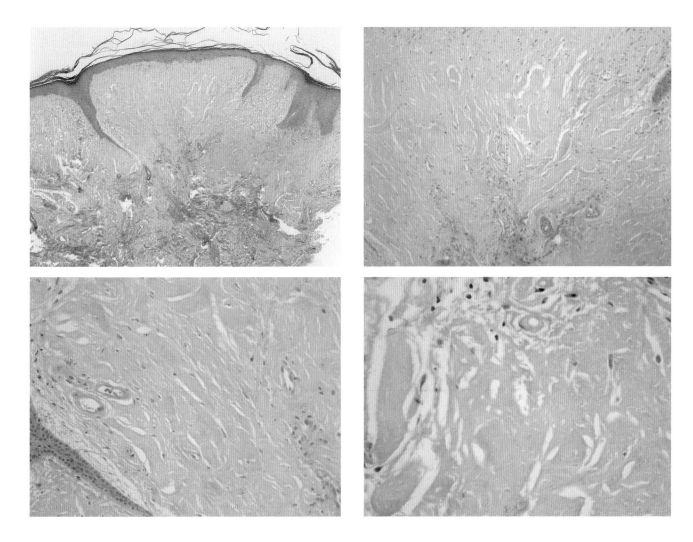

- Dermal material that is pink and amorphous and fills the upper half of the dermis
- Early lesions have pink material around vessels

Erythropoietic protoporphyria

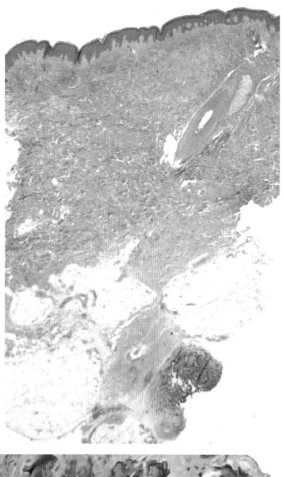

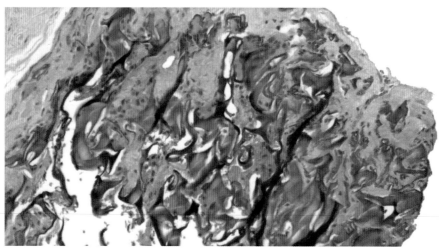

• Dermal material that is bluish, curvy, and ribbon-like

Gel foam

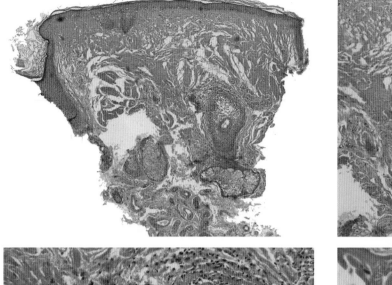
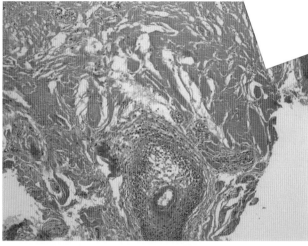
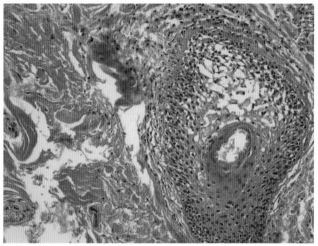
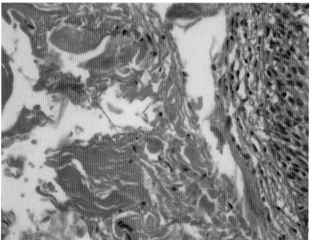

- Dermal material that is pink and amorphous, often filling the dermis full-thickness
- May be perpendicular to epidermis and around adnexae and vessels

Lipoid proteinosis

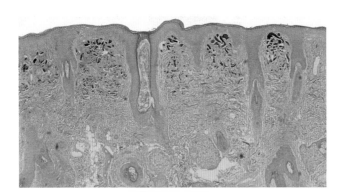
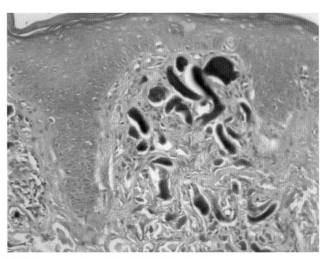
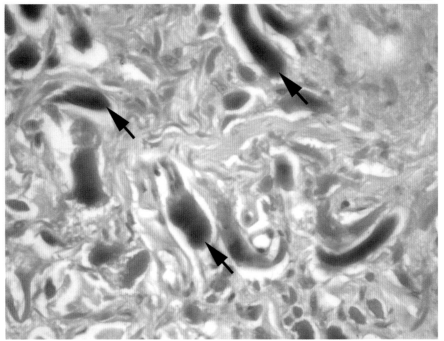

• Dermal material that is banana-shaped and brown–orange
  (arrows)

Ochronosis

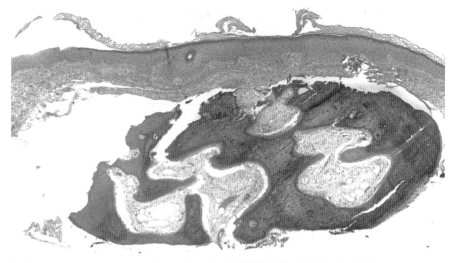

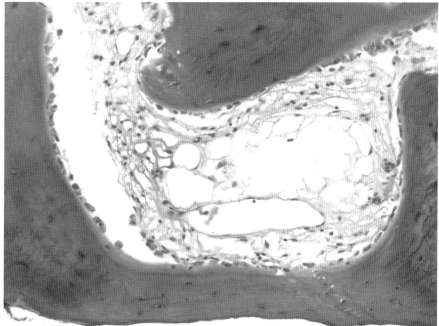

- Dermal material
- Bright, dense pink trabeculae with nuclei with haloes around them (osteocytes)
- Pilomatricomas can be ossified

Osteoma cutis

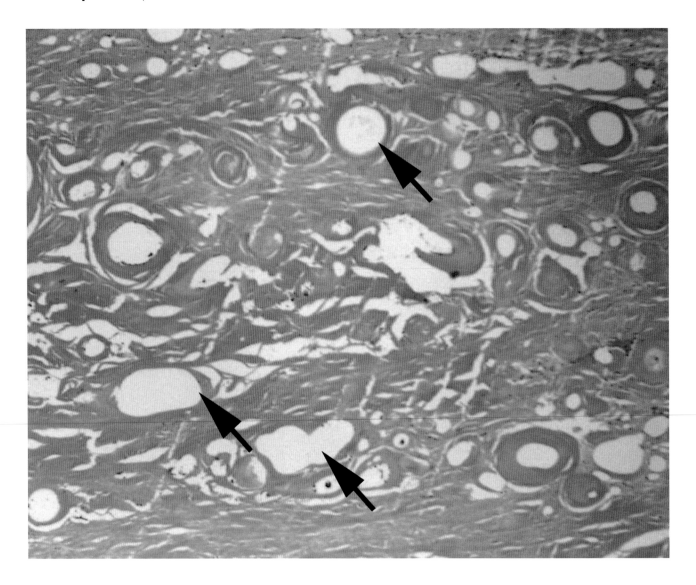

- Dermal material that is lost during processing and is "seen" as irregularly shaped circular spaces (arrows)
- Dark pink sclerotic stroma
- Swiss-cheese appearance

Paraffinoma

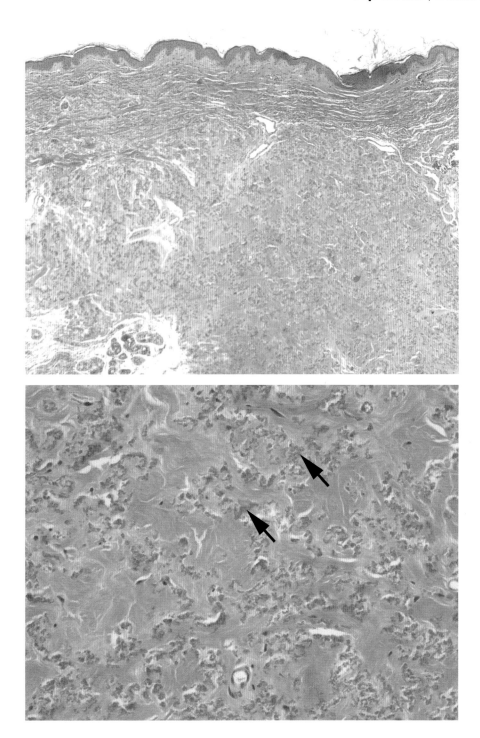

- Dermal material that is blue and squiggly (arrows)
- Sometimes the corkscrew fibers are calcified

Pseudoxanthoma elasticum

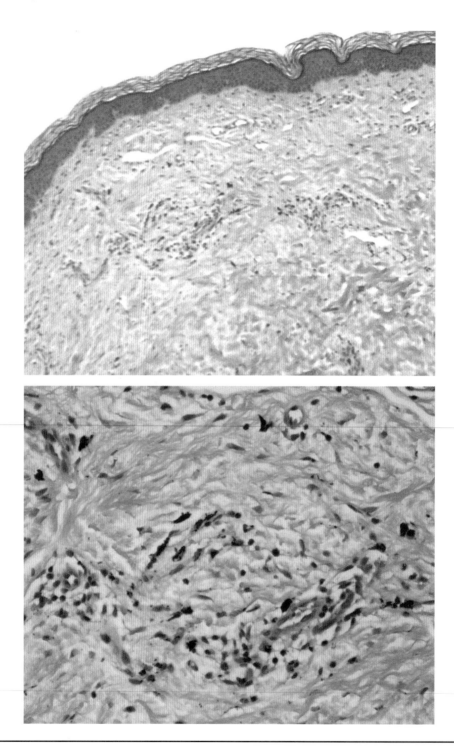

- Dermal material that is black (most commonly) and is free in
  the dermis as well as within macrophages

Tattoo

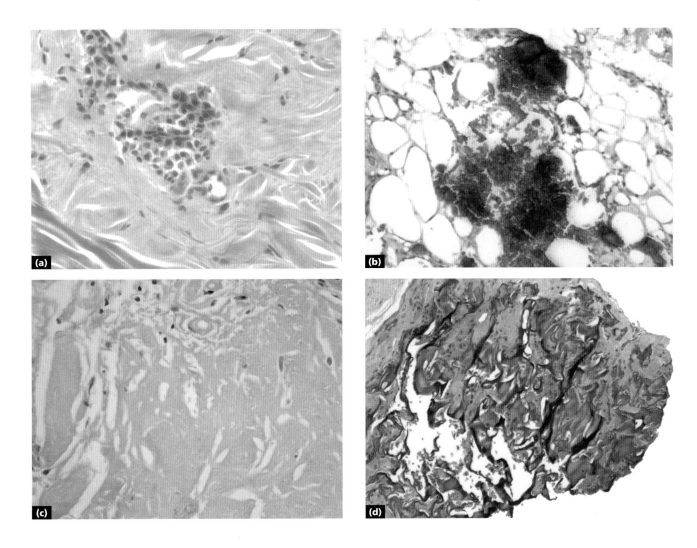

Dermal material

- **a** Amyloidosis, nodular: amorphous pink material with plasma cells
- **b** Calcinosis cutis: blue–purple chunks
- **c** Erythropoietic protoporphyria: amorphous pink material around vessels and in upper dermis
- **d** Gel foam: blue interconnected ribbons

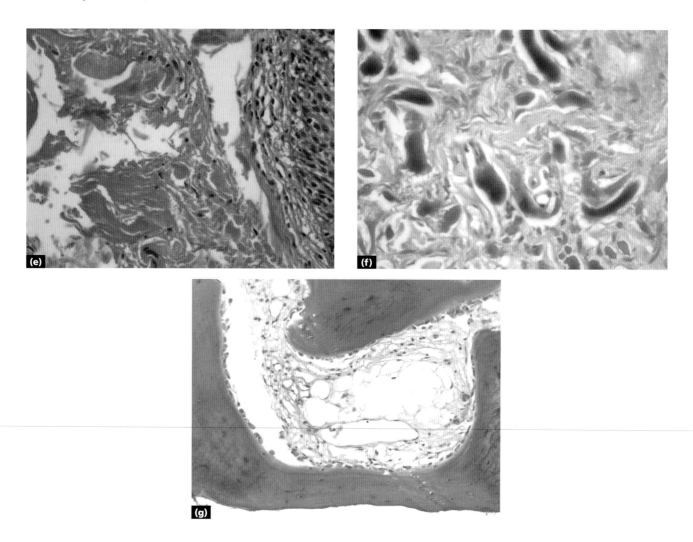

Dermal material (cont.)

- **e** Lipoid proteinosis: amorphous pink material filling the entire dermis; often around adnexae
- **f** Ochronosis: brown–orange banana shapes
- **g** Osteoma cutis: well-defined pink shapes with nuclei

Key differences

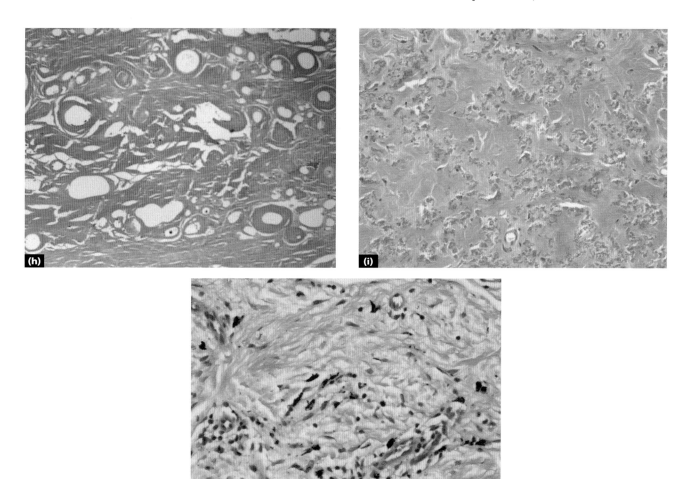

Dermal material (cont.)

- **h** Paraffinoma: irregular circular spaces like Swiss cheese
- **i** Pseudoxanthoma elasticum: squiggly blue lines
- **j** Tattoo: black particles within macrophages and free in dermis

Key differences

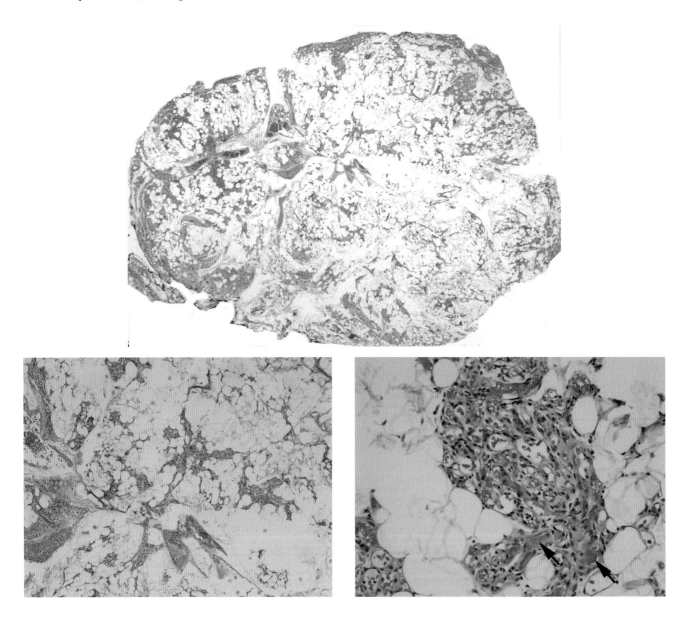

- Change in the fat
- Normal-appearing adipocytes in lobules with an increased number of small vessels, some containing fibrin (arrows)

Angiolipoma

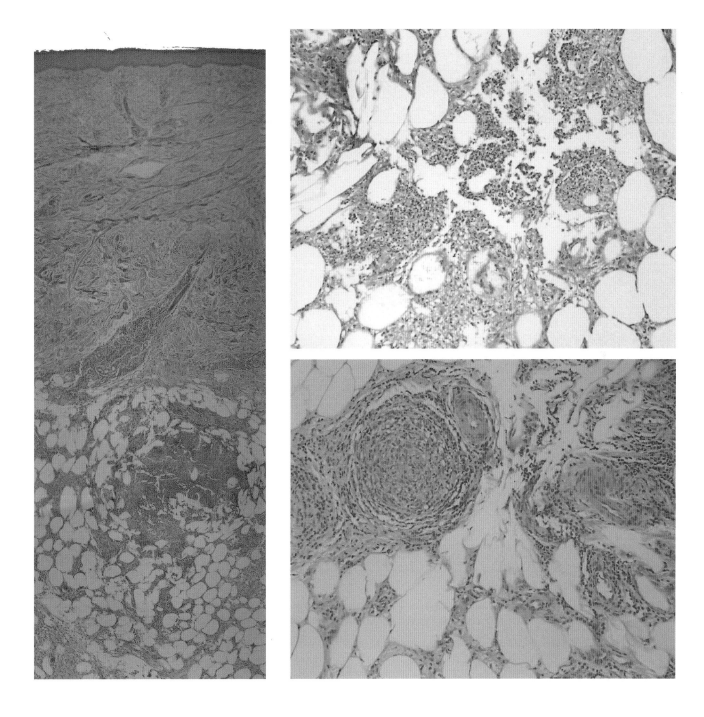

- Change in the fat
- Lobular panniculitis with mixed inflammation (histiocytes, lymphocytes, neutrophils)
- Inflammation around vessels (vasculitis) in the septae
- "Panniculitis > vasculitis"; compare with polyarteritis nodosa

Erythema induratum

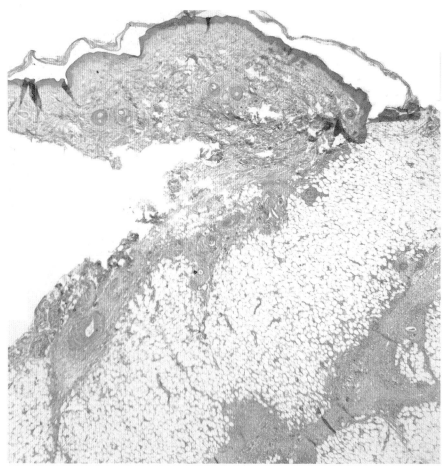

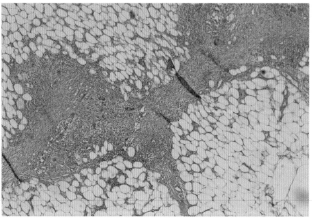

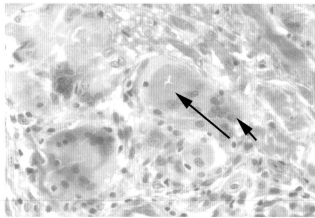

- Change in the fat
- Septal panniculitis with thickened septae between lobules of adipocytes

- Septae contain giant cells (short arrow)
- Early lesions may have neutrophils, eosinophils
- Miescher's radial granuloma may be seen (long arrow)

Erythema nodosum

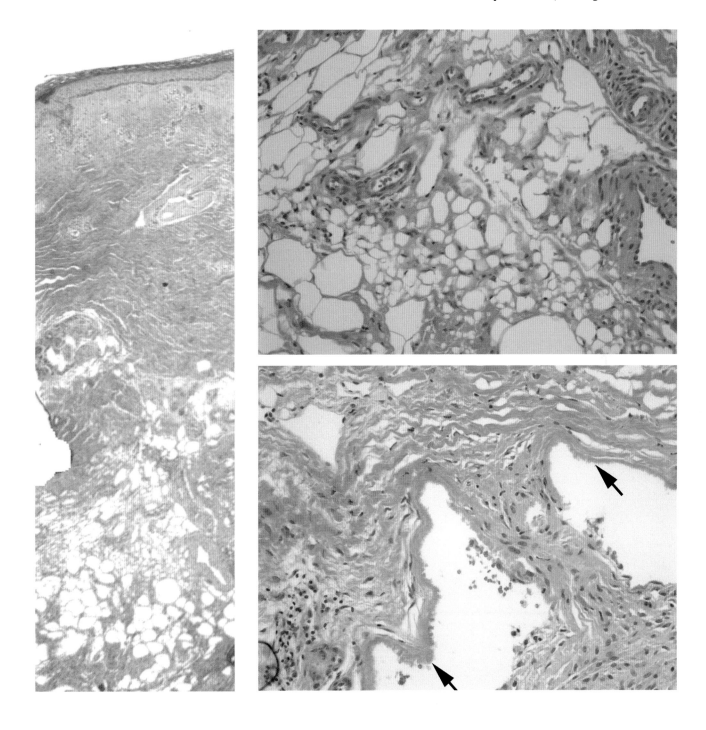

- Change in the fat
- Individual adipocytes are lost and replaced by arabesques of pink, ruffled membranes (lipomembranous fat necrosis) (arrows)

Lipodermatosclerosis

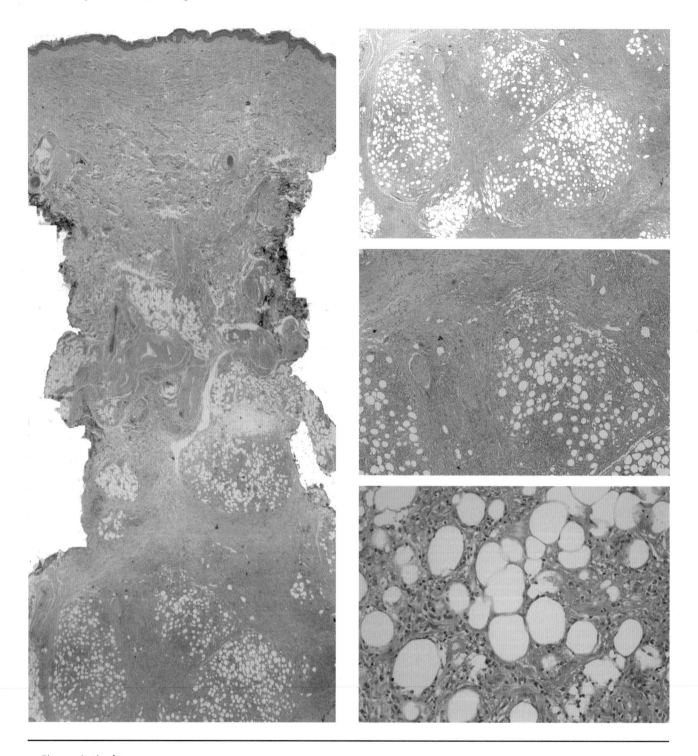

- Change in the fat
- Lymphoplasmacytic infiltrate (lobular panniculitis)
- Lymphoid follicles may be present
- Fibrinoid (hyaline) necrosis of fat
- Later stages show hyalinization of fat (hyaline sclerosis)

Lupus profundus

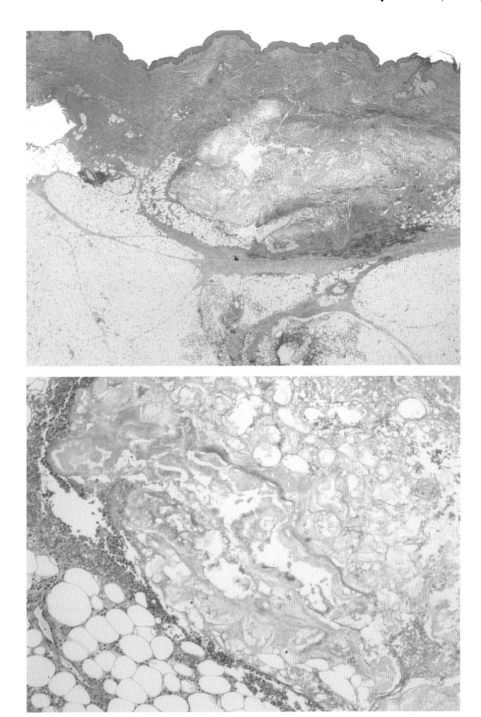

- Change in the fat
- Necrosis of the fat with "ghost-like" shadows of fat cells remaining
- Calcification/neutrophils/eosinophils may be present
- Septal vessels are inflamed

Pancreatic fat necrosis

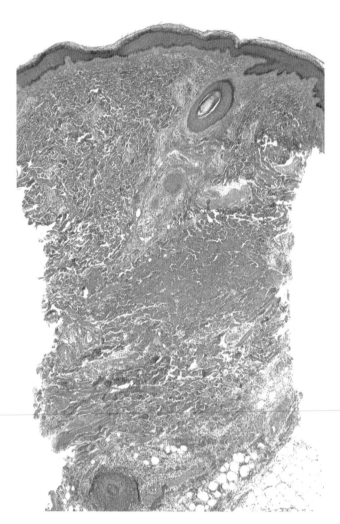

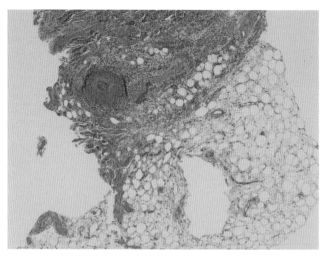

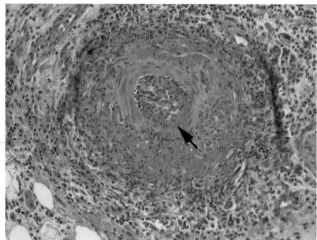

- Change in the fat
- Septal panniculitis
- Often at dermal–subcutis junction, a large vessel is involved with inflammation (vasculitis) (arrow)

- "Vasculitis > panniculitis"; compare with erythema induratum

Polyarteritis nodosa

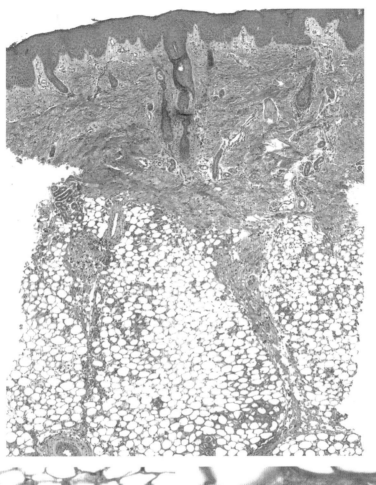

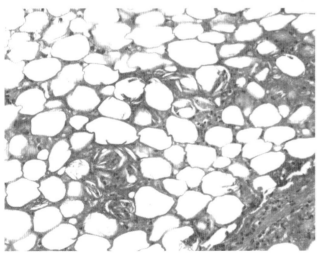

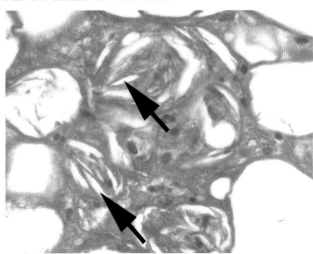

- Change in the fat
- Lobular panniculitis
- Inflammation and radial crystalline shapes (arrows) within fat lobules

- Note that post-steroid panniculitis can look the same
- Note that sclerema neonatorum also has crystalline shapes but lacks inflammation

Subcutaneous fat necrosis of the newborn

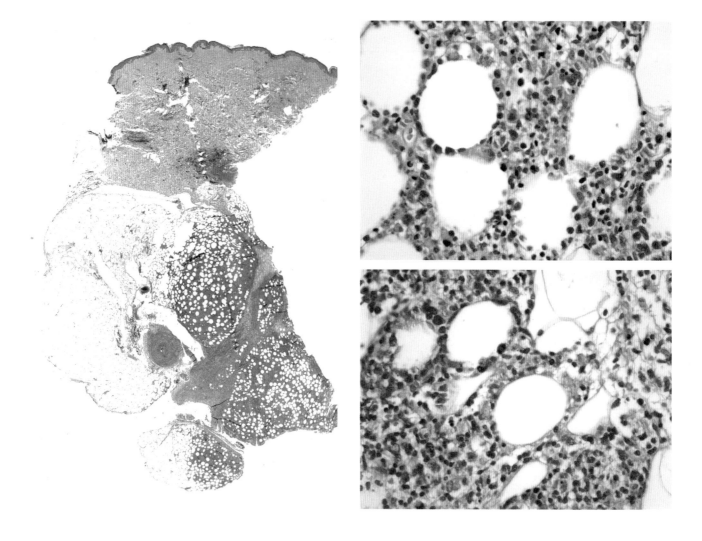

- Change in the fat
- Lobular involvement of inflammation
- Atypical lymphocytes rim fat cells

Figures are courtesy of Antonio Subtil, MD.

Subcutaneous T-cell lymphoma

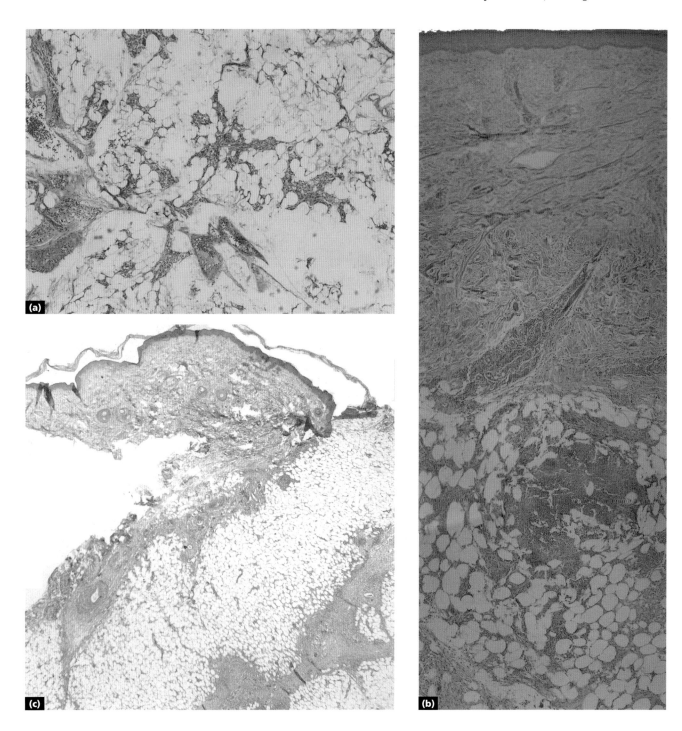

Change in the fat
- **a** Angiolipoma: normal adipocytes, increased numbers of vessels with fibrin
- **b** Erythema induratum: vasculitis and lobular mixed inflammation, "panniculitis > vasculitis"

- **c** Erythema nodosum: septal thickening with giant cells (sometimes eosinophils)

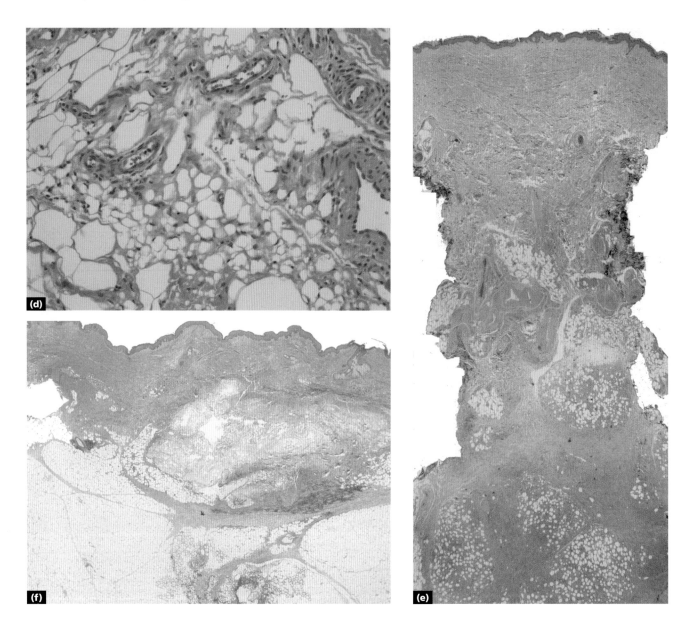

Change in the fat (cont.)

- **d** Lipodermatosclerosis: pink arabesques of membranes replacing adipocytes
- **e** Lupus profundus: hyaline fat necrosis, lymphocytic lobular infiltrate
- **f** Pancreatic fat necrosis: ghost-like necrosis of fat, +/– calcification

Key differences

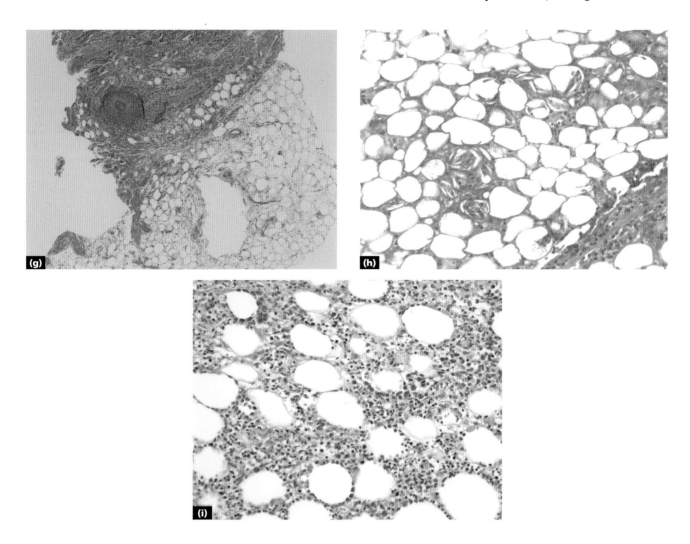

Change in the fat (cont.)

- **g** Polyarteritis nodosa: vasculitis of a medium-sized vessel, often at dermal–subcutis junction, "vasculitis > panniculitis"
- **h** Subcutaneous fat necrosis of the newborn: crystalline shapes and inflammation within fat lobules
- **i** Subcutaneous T-cell lymphoma: rimming of adipocytes with atypical lymphocytes

Figure (i) is courtesy of Antonio Subtil, MD.

Key differences

3 Cell Type

- Clear, 177
- Melanocytic, 194
- Spindle, 203
- Giant, 216

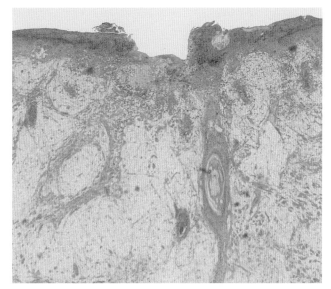

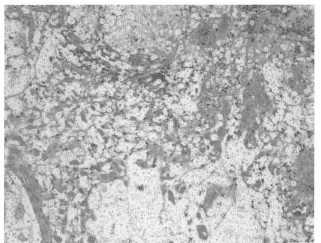
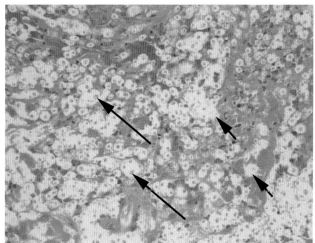

- Clear "cells"
- The organisms (long arrows) are surrounded by capsules, which are seen in sections as clear spaces (short arrows)

Cryptococcosis, gelatinous

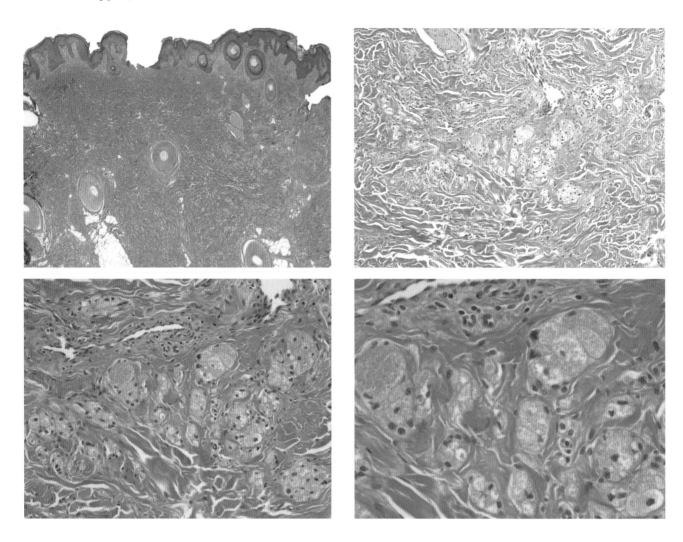

- "Clear" cells
- Epidermis may be acanthotic or display pseudoepitheliomatous hyperplasia
- Cells are polygonal to oval and contain a granular pink material (phagolysosomes)
- Large granules are surrounded by haloes

Granular cell tumor

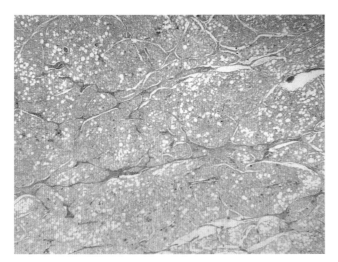
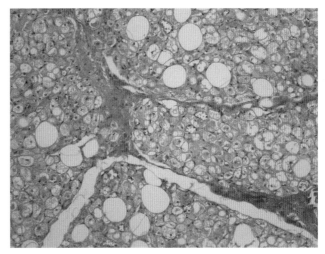
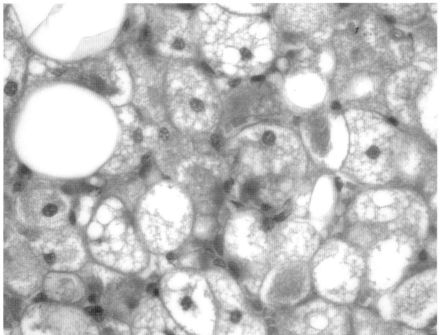

- "Clear" cells
- Cells are adipocytes that are so-called "mulberry" cells, with a net-like vacuolar pattern around the nuclei

Hibernoma

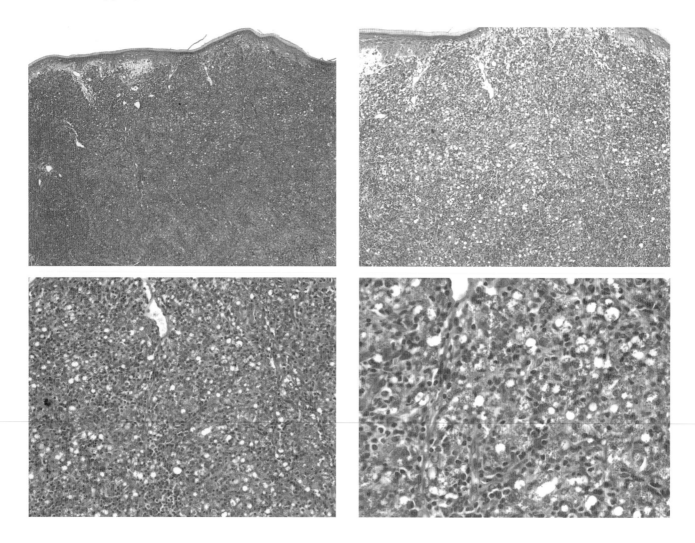

- "Clear" cells
- Cells are macrophages that contain the organisms

Leishmaniasis

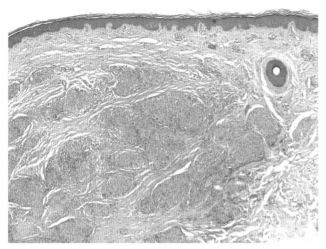
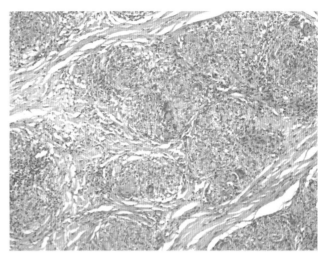
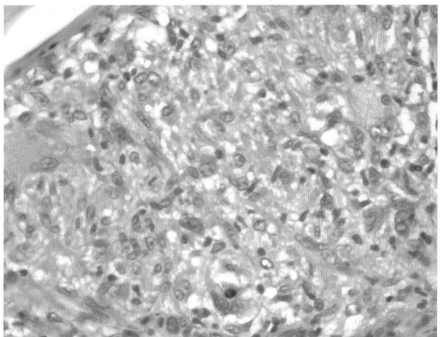

- "Clear" cells
- Cells are histiocytes ("Virchow cells") that look subtly foamy and are filled with organisms (seen with special stains)
- Vacuoles with clusters of organisms (globi)

- On low power, the histiocytes are arranged in linear configurations
- Grenz zone present
- Nerves may appear thickened

Lepromatous leprosy

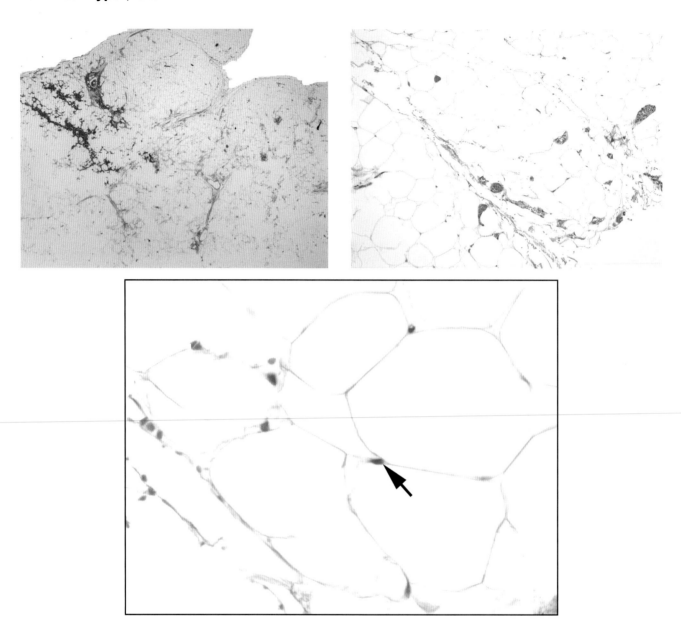

- "Clear" cells
- Cells are adipocytes, with a peripheral, compressed nucleus (arrow)

Lipoma

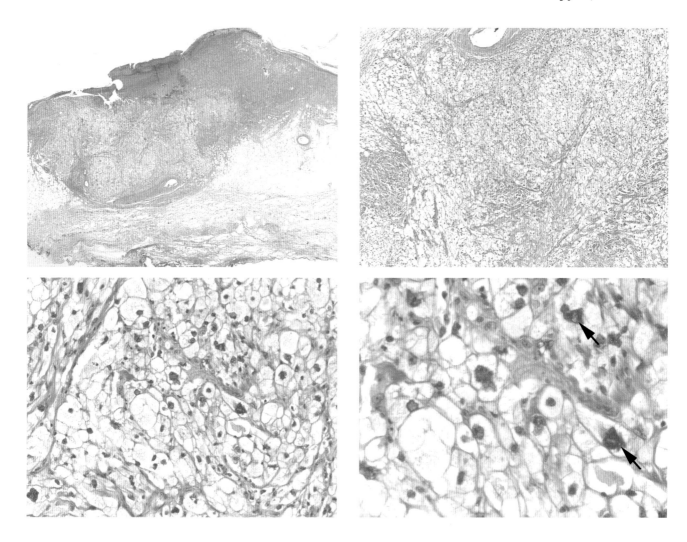

- "Clear" cells
- Cells are melanocytes that have clear/foamy cytoplasm
- Cells have atypical nuclei (arrows)

- Special stains are generally necessary to confirm the diagnosis
- Look for foci of conventional melanoma or a junctional component

Melanoma, balloon cell

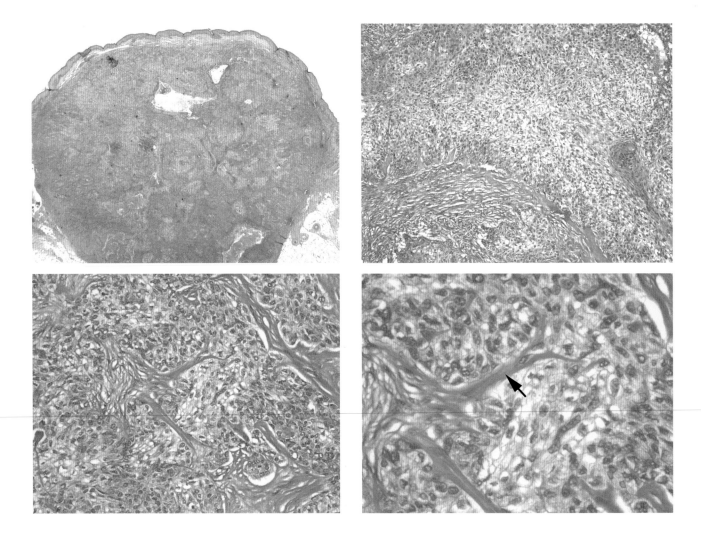

- "Clear" cells
- Cells are arranged in lobules with areas of ductal differentiation
- Hyalinized collagen often present (arrows)

Nodular hidradenoma

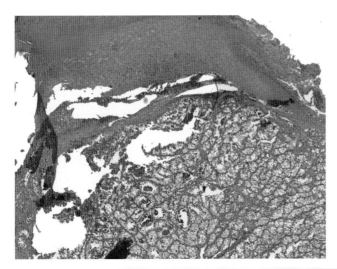
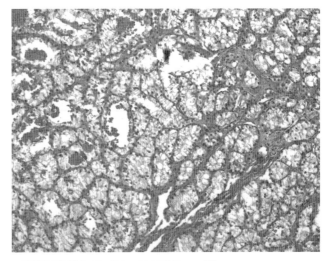
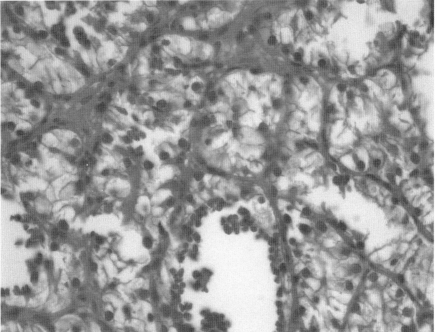

- "Clear" cells
- Often in cords, islands, or pseudoglandular structures
- Cells are of renal origin and are surrounded by prominent blood vessels/extravasated erythrocytes

Renal cell carcinoma

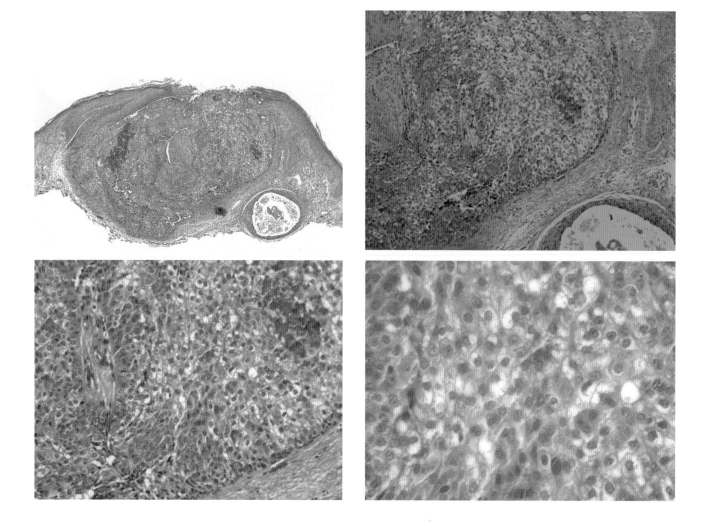

- "Clear" cells
- Cells are sebocytes with spiky/scalloped nuclei bordered by several layers of basaloid cells
- Generally on low power there is a downward lobular proliferation from the epidermis

Sebaceous adenoma

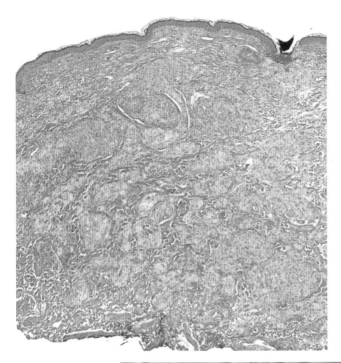

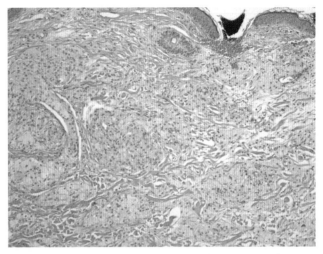

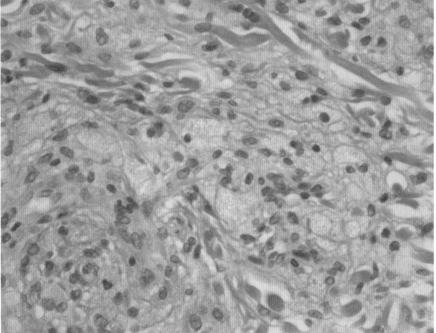

- "Clear" cells
- Cells are foamy histiocytes (filled with lipid), arranged in between collagen bundles
- Often a thin epidermis (eyelid skin)
- Vellus hairs may be present (eyelid skin)

Xanthelasma

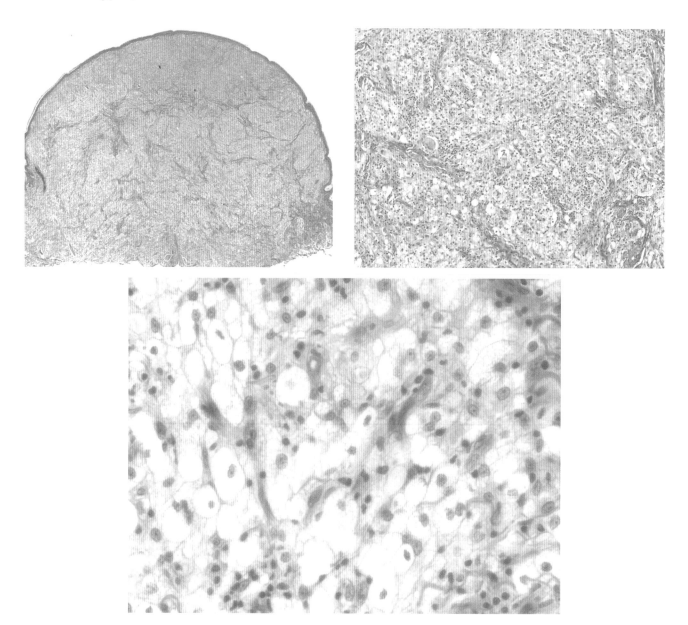

- "Clear" cells
- Cells are histiocytes, arranged in a well-circumscribed mass in the upper dermis
- Touton giant cells and eosinophils often seen

Xanthogranuloma (older lesion)

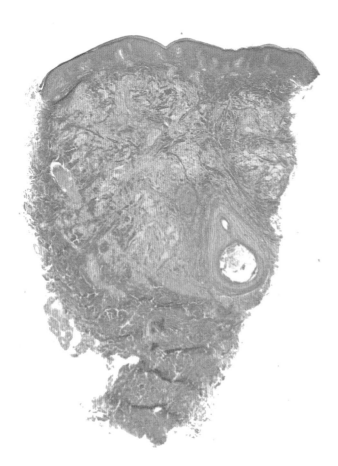

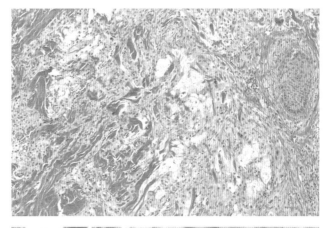

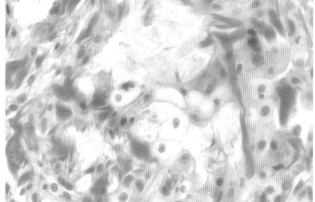

- "Clear" cells
- Cells are foamy histiocytes (filled with lipid), in clusters in the dermis
- Free lipid is present in eruptive xanthomas

Xanthoma

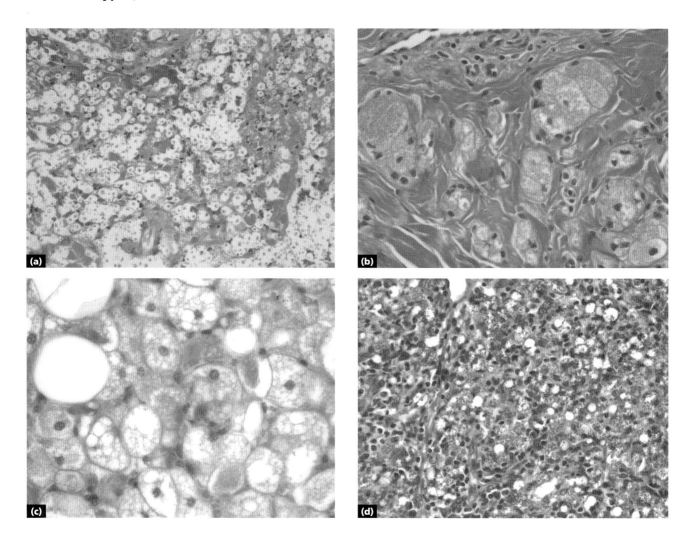

"Clear cells"

- **a** Cryptococcosis, gelatinous: clear spaces representing the capsule of the organism

- **b** Granular cell tumor: cells with grainy cytoplasm, small and large
- **c** Hibernoma: cells with net-like vacuolated cytoplasm
- **d** Leishmaniasis: macrophages filled with organisms

Key differences

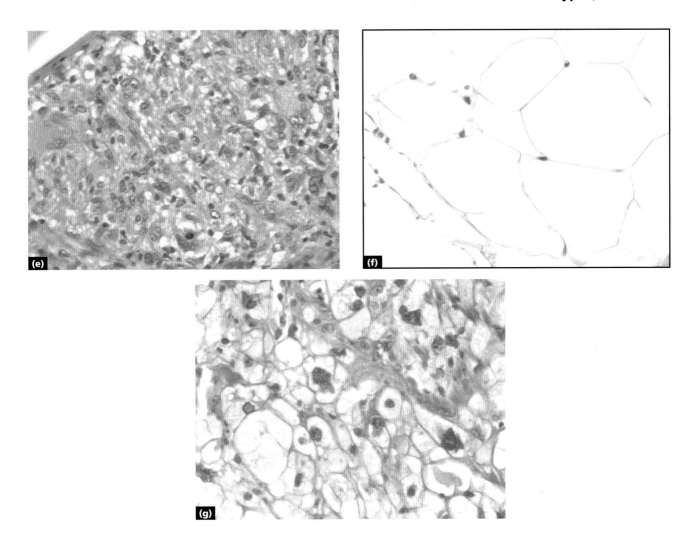

"Clear cells" (cont.)

- **e** Lepromatous leprosy: histiocytes filled with organisms; linear arrangement on low power
- **f** Lipoma: clear adipocytes; peripheral nuclei
- **g** Melanoma, balloon cell: atypical nuclei with clear cytoplasm

Key differences

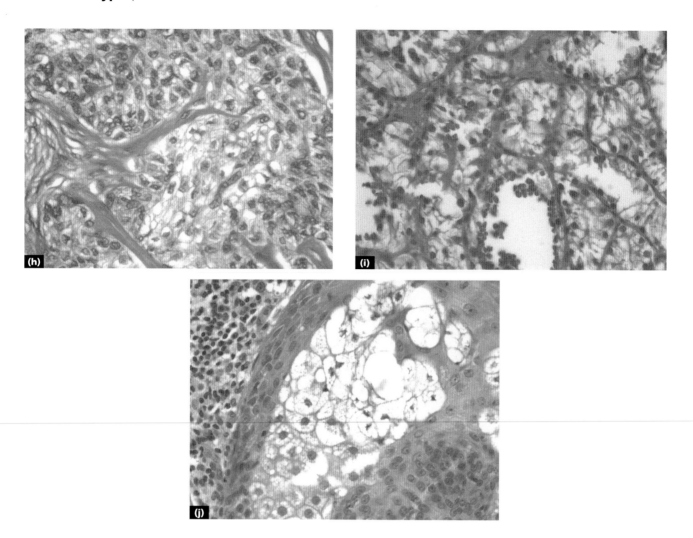

"Clear cells" (cont.)

- **h** Nodular hidradenoma: clear cells with interspersed ducts and hyalinized collagen
- **i** Renal cell carcinoma: clear cells with extravasated erythrocytes
- **j** Sebaceous adenoma: clear sebocytes with star-shaped nuclei with a rim of basaloid cells

Key differences

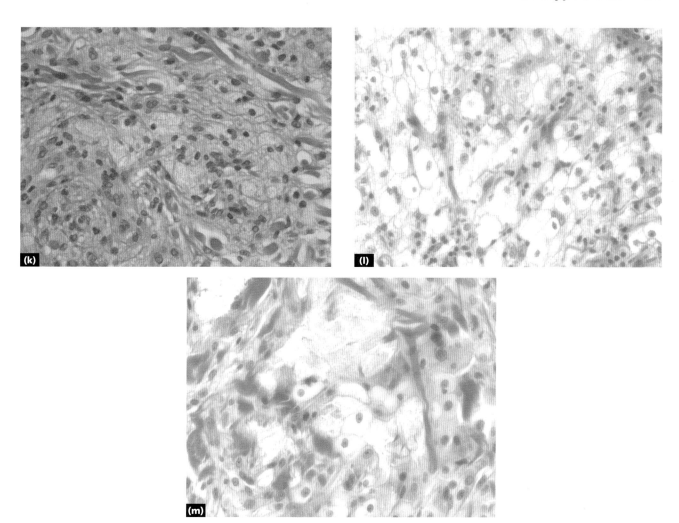

"Clear cells" (cont.)

- **k** Xanthelasma: foamy cells interspersed in eyelid skin
- **l** Xanthogranuloma: foamy cells with some Touton cells
- **m** Xanthoma: foamy cells and extracellular lipid

Key differences

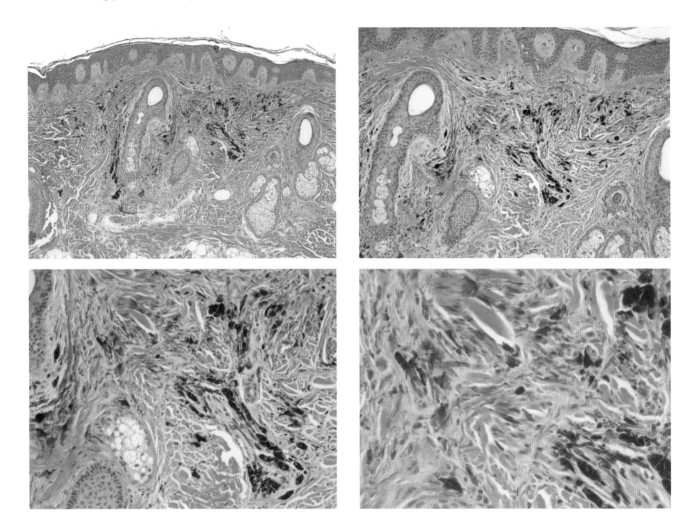

- Melanocytic cells
- Cells are small and spindled/dendritic with occasional cells containing melanin pigment
- Dermis often hyalinized
- Melanophages often present

Blue nevus

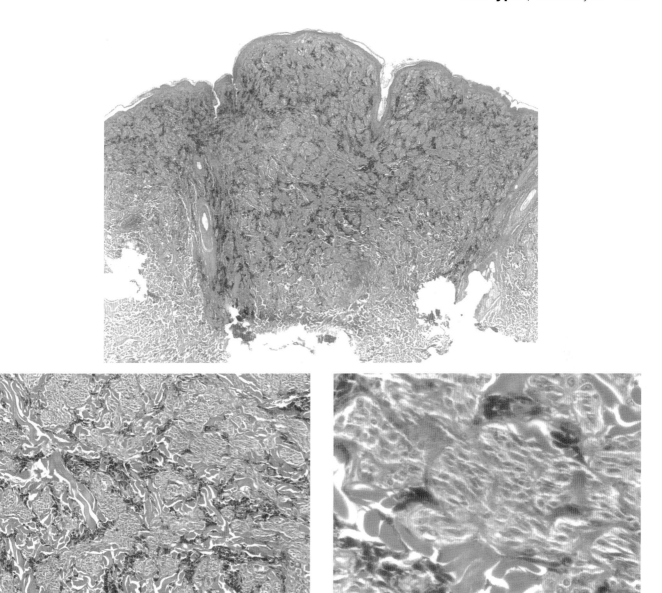

- Melanocytic cells
- Epithelioid melanocytes are admixed with or bordered by uniformly distributed melanophages
- Pattern on low power is wedge-shaped (often centered around a follicle)

Deep penetrating nevus

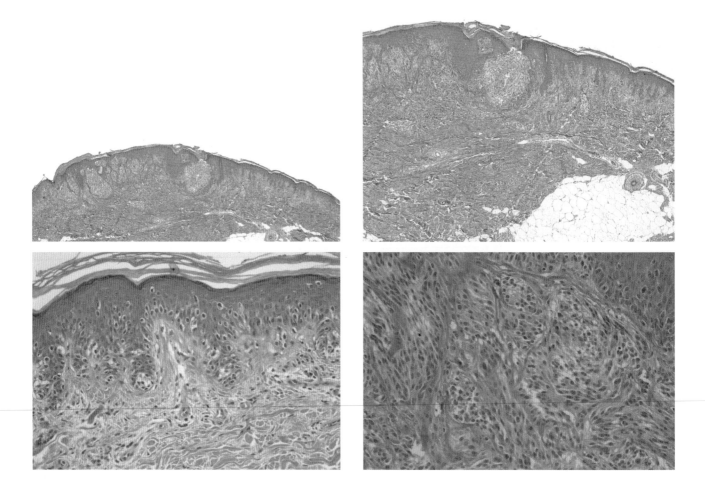

- Melanocytic cells
- Cells are confluent at the junction with irregularly sized nests, scattered high and low within the epidermis
- Atypical cells and mitoses in epidermal and dermal nests

Melanoma

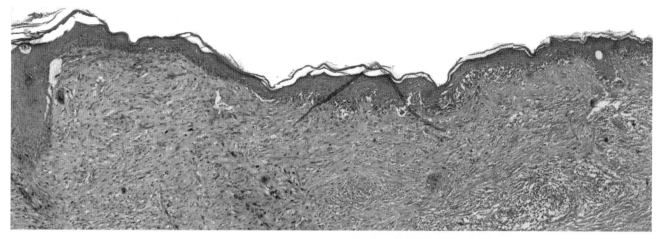

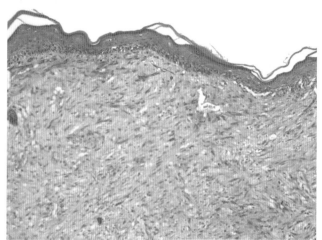
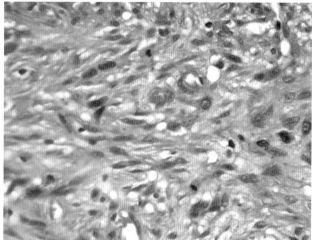

- Melanocytic cells
- Cells are spindled and arranged in bundles infiltrating through collagen
- Cells are atypical
- Often overlying in situ melanoma changes in epidermis

Melanoma, desmoplastic

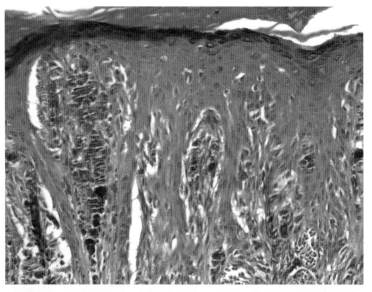

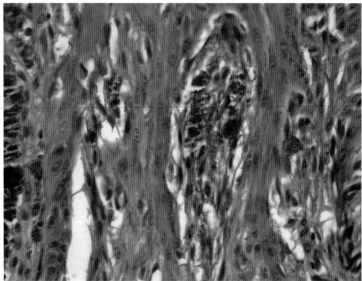

- Melanocytic cells
- Pigmented spindle cells are arranged in vertical fascicles in
  the base of the epidermis

Pigmented spindle cell nevus of Reed

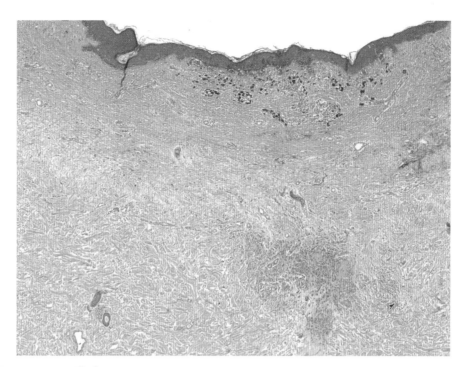

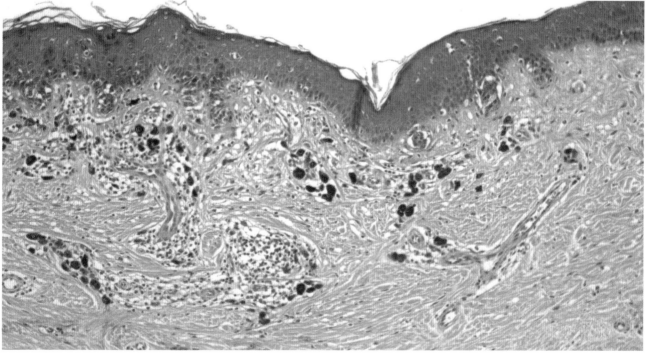

- Melanocytic cells
- Cells are in irregularly shaped nests, sometimes confluent,
  confined to the area above a dermal scar
- Predominantly junctional involvement

Recurrent nevus

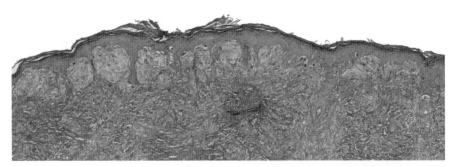

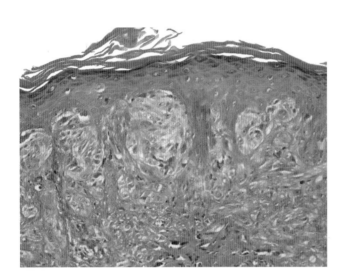

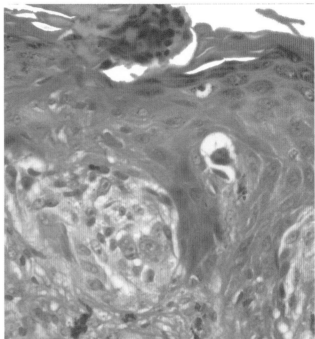

- Melanocytic cells, spindled and epithelioid
- Cells are in vertical fascicles within the epidermis ("school of fish")
- Well circumscribed and symmetric
- Kamino bodies
- Clefting above nests
- Cells are atypical but all resemble each other

Spitz nevus

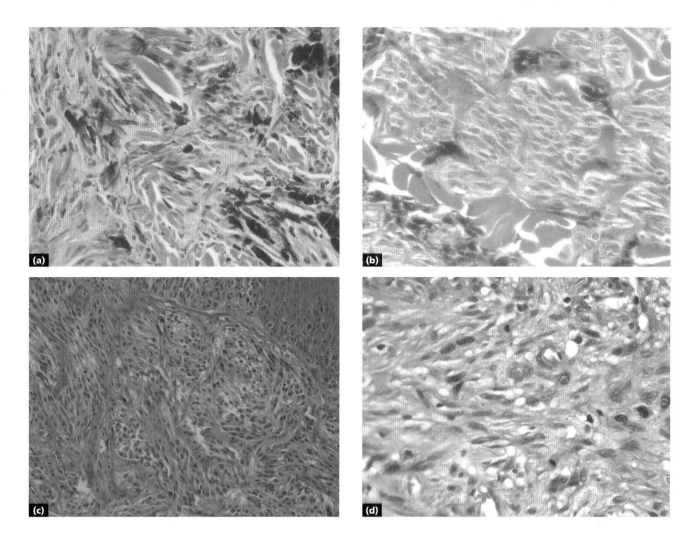

Melanocytic cells

- **a** Blue nevus: finely pigmented spindle/dendritic cells within the dermis
- **b** Deep penetrating nevus: wedge-shaped epithelioid melanocytes admixed with melanophages
- **c** Melanoma: atypical cells in epidermis and dermis, asymmetric, dermal mitoses
- **d** Melanoma, desmoplastic: atypical spindle cells infiltrating through collagen

Key differences

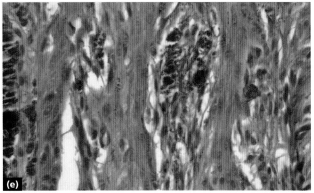

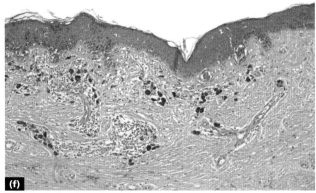

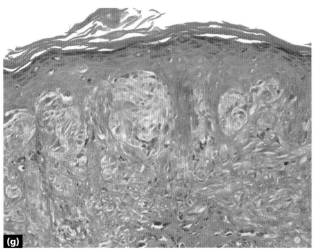

Melanocytic cells (cont.)

- **e** Pigmented spindle cell nevus of Reed: vertically arranged pigmented cells in base of epidermis

- **f** Recurrent nevus: irregular nests of pigmented cells above a scar
- **g** Spitz nevus: vertically arranged epithelioid and spindle cells; symmetric

Key differences

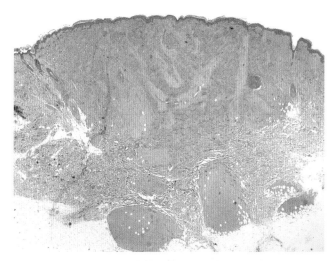
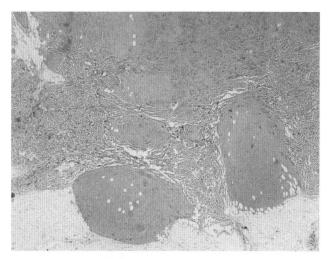
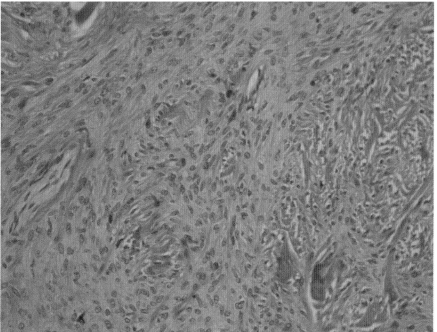

- Spindle cells (which also appear rounded when fascicles are cut cross-wise) (so-called biphasic pattern)
- Often bulbous into the deep dermis
- Scattered melanin pigment within the cells

Blue nevus, cellular

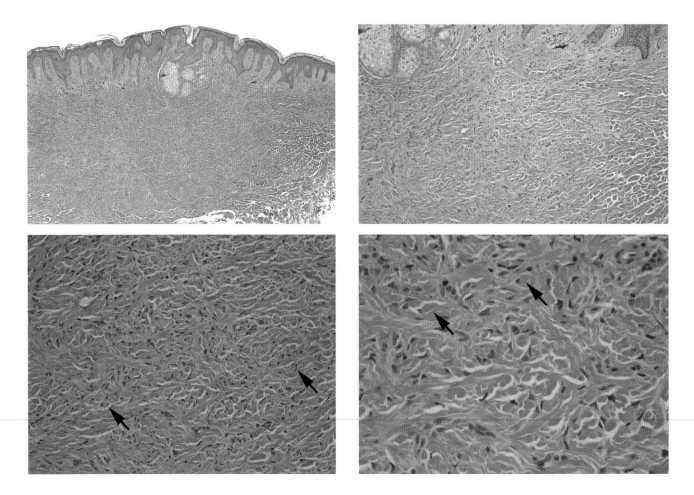

- Spindle cells in a "busy dermis"
- Epidermis often acanthotic and pigmented
- Cells entrap collagen at the periphery (arrows)

Dermatofibroma

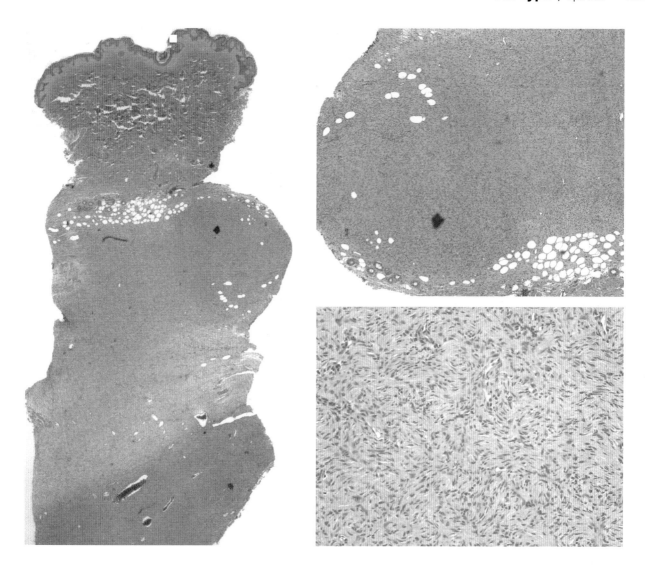

- Spindle cells filling dermis
- Cells are monomorphous and arranged in a storiform
  (cartwheel) pattern
- Infiltration into the fat in layered or honeycomb pattern

Dermatofibrosarcoma protuberans

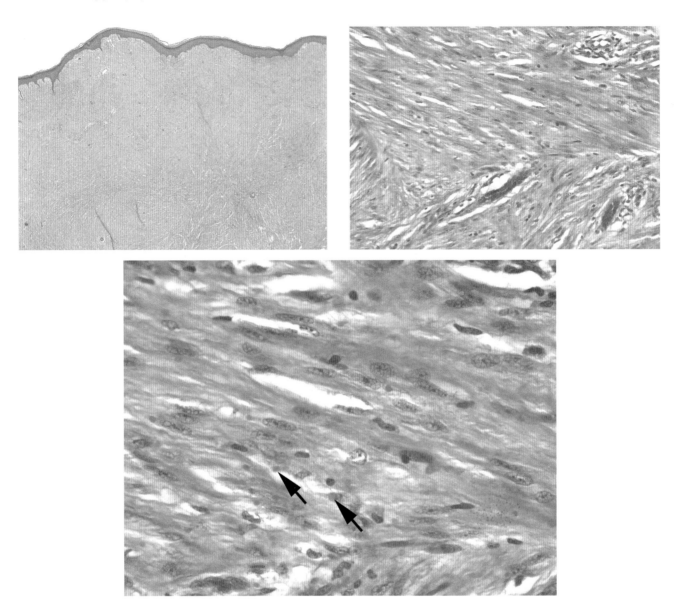

- Spindle cells
- Cells have round pink cytoplasmic inclusions (arrows)
- Cells are arranged in long fascicles

Infantile digital fibromatosis

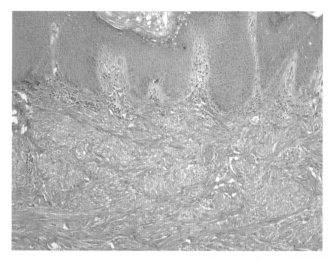

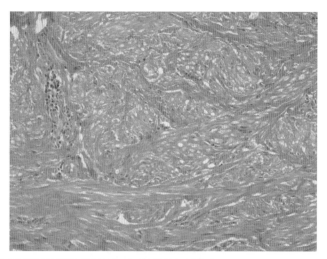

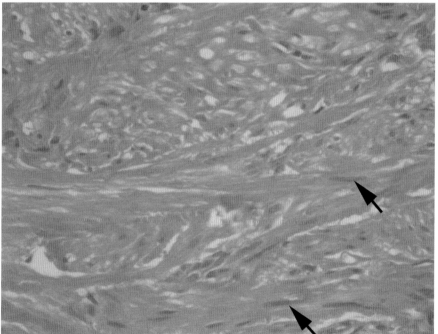

- Spindle cells
- Cells are arranged in fascicles which intersect at 90 degree angles
- Spindle cells cut longitudinally show "cigar-shaped" nuclei (arrows)

- Cells cut in cross-section have perinuclear vacuoles around round nuclei
- Note that normal nipple has small bundles of smooth muscle cells (same appearance as an accessory nipple, see p. 4)

Leiomyoma

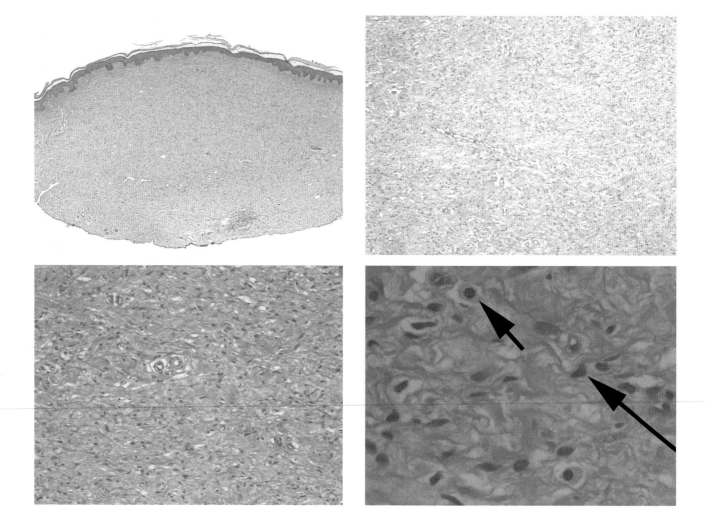

- Spindle cells
- Cells have thin, wavy nuclei (long arrow), looks like "shredded carrot"
- Bubble-gum pink stroma

- Scattered mast cells (short arrow)
- Not encapsulated

Neurofibroma

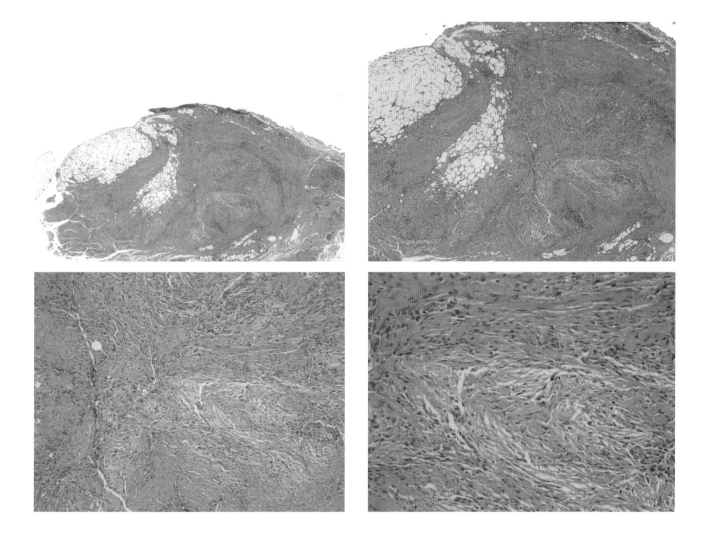

- Spindle cells
- Myxoid areas of elongated cells with oval nuclei with tapered ends and elongated cytoplasm ("tissue-culture" fibroblasts)
- Extravasated erythrocytes

- Mitoses may be seen
- Radial arrangement of blood vessels at periphery
- Deep tumor, often no epidermis present

Nodular fasciitis

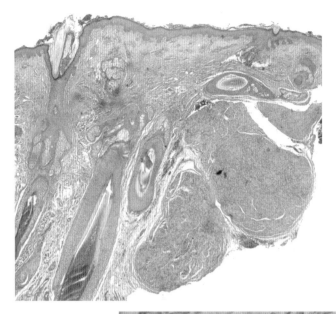
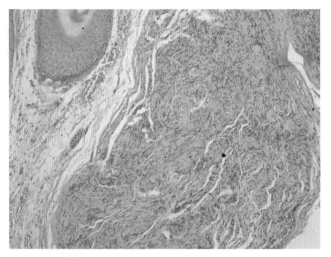
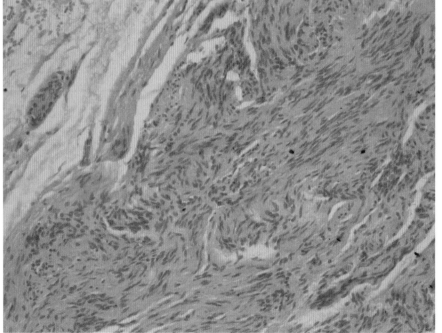

- Spindle cells
- Cells are arranged in fascicles with characteristic clefting
- Not truly encapsulated

Palisaded encapsulated neuroma

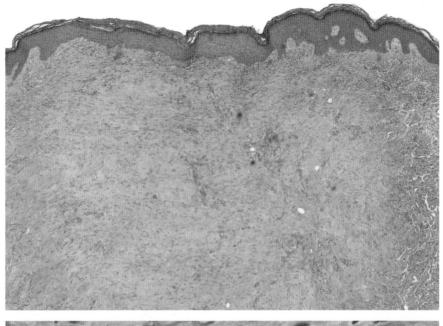

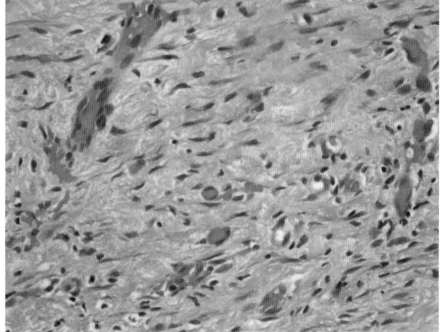

- Spindle cells
- Cells are arranged parallel to epidermis
- Vessels oriented perpendicular to epidermal surface

Scar

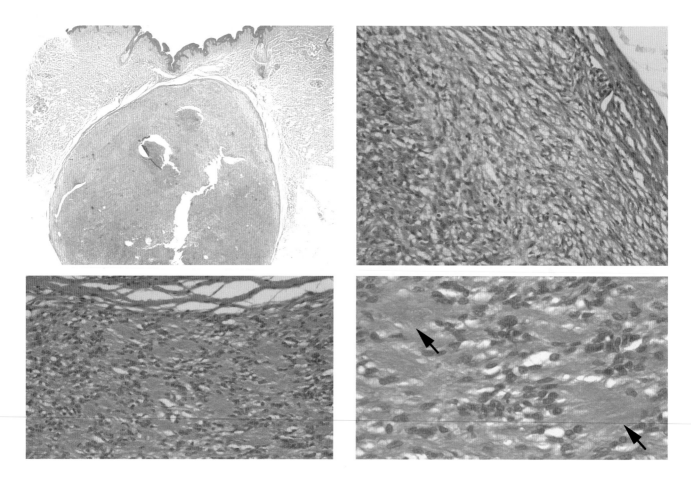

- Spindle cells
- Antoni A areas – cellular
- Antoni B areas – myxoid
- Verocay bodies (arrows) – palisaded arrangement of nuclei around a central pink area of collagen

- Encapsulated
- Vascular spaces may be very dilated
- Often a deep tumor with no epidermis present

Schwannoma

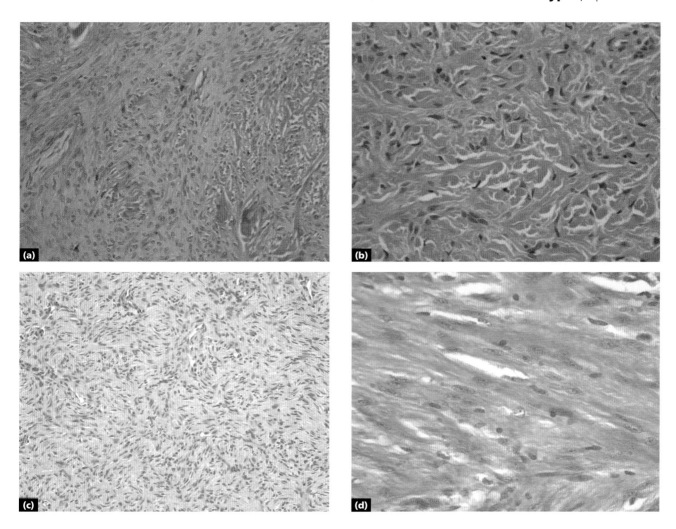

Spindle cells

- **a** Blue nevus, cellular: bulbous projection into deeper dermis, some cells have melanin pigment
- **b** Dermatofibroma: collagen entrapment at periphery, epidermal acanthosis
- **c** Dermatofibrosarcoma protuberans: monomorphous cells in cartwheel arrangement; infiltration into fat
- **d** Infantile digital fibromatosis: bright pink cytoplasmic inclusions

Key differences

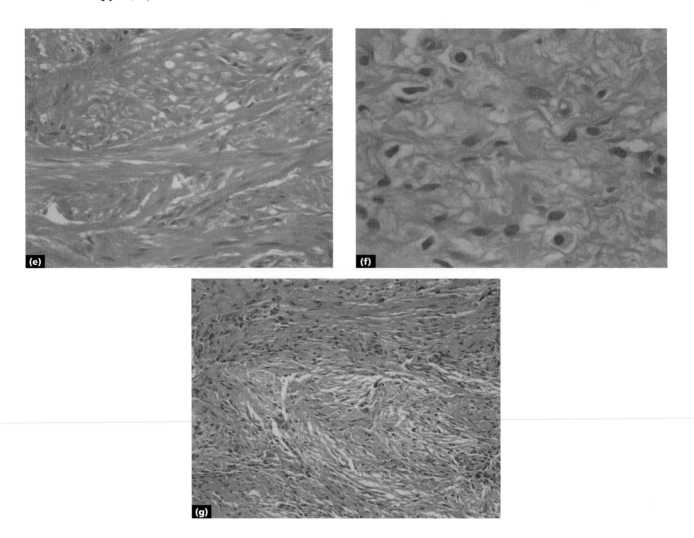

Spindle cells (cont.)

- **e** Leiomyoma: cigar-shaped nuclei in long fascicles
- **f** Neurofibroma: wavy nuclei, mast cells, bubble-gum pink stroma
- **g** Nodular fasciitis: tissue-culture fibroblasts, extravasated erythrocytes, often deep in the fat

Key differences

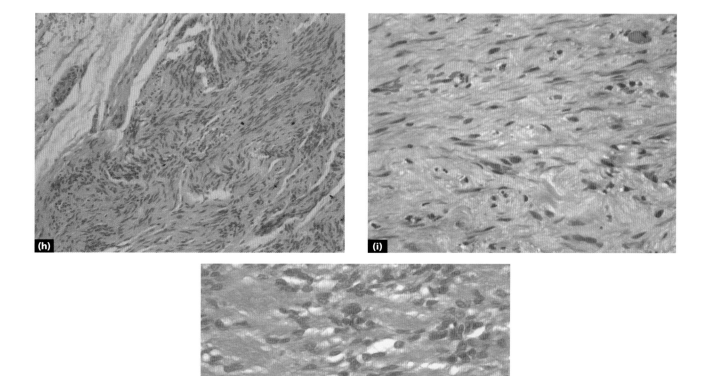

Spindle cells (cont.)

- **h** Palisaded encapsulated neuroma: clefts between collections of spindle cells with nuclear palisading
- **i** Scar: spindle cells arranged parallel to epidermal surface
- **j** Schwannoma: Verocay bodies, myxoid areas, encapsulated

Key differences

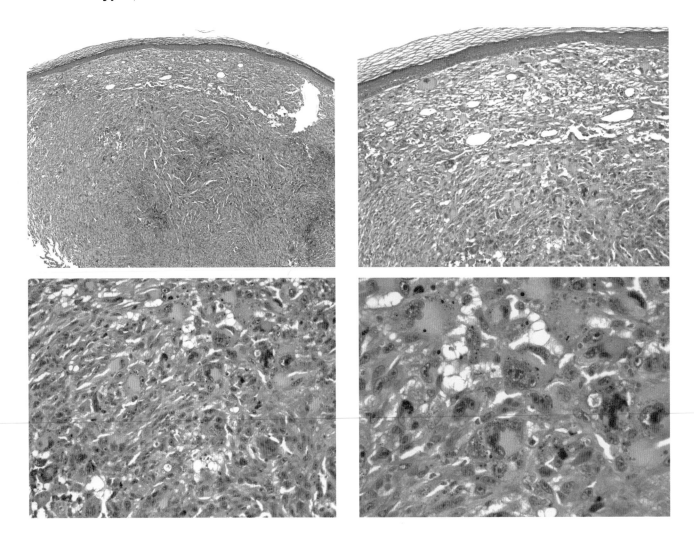

- Giant cells with bizarre nuclei
- Cells are atypical
- Mitoses
- Often a grenz zone above the atypical cells and solar elastosis flanking the atypical cells

Atypical fibroxanthoma

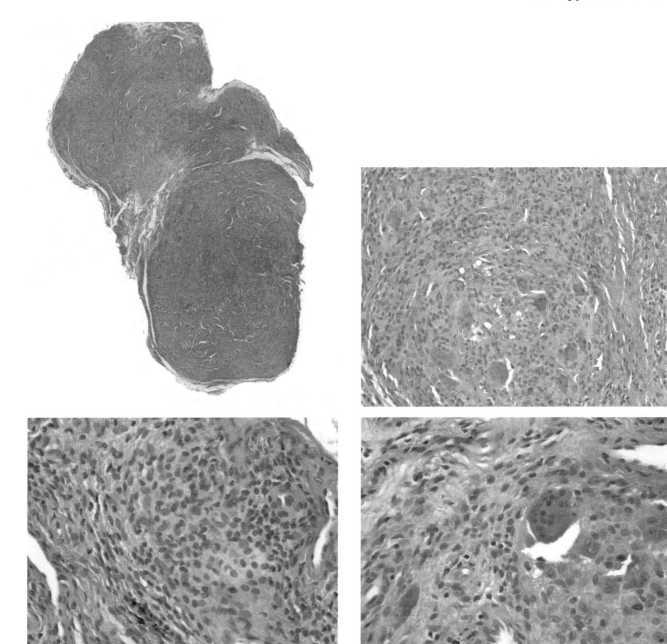

- Giant cells of osteoclastic type (nuclei arranged haphazardly on one side of the cell)
- Nuclei of giant cells resemble the nuclei of adjacent histiocytes
- Hemosiderophages
- Often a deep tumor (no epidermis present)

Giant cell tumor of tendon sheath

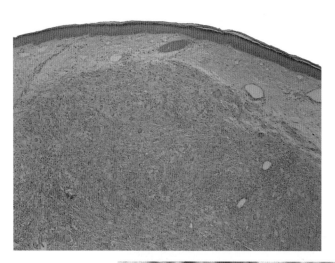
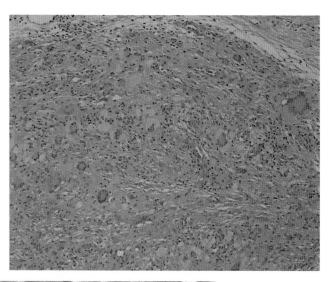
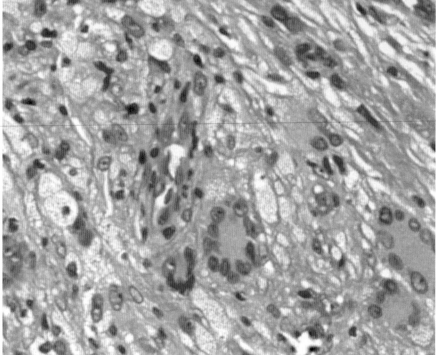

- Touton giant cells (wreath of nuclei with pink center and foamy cytoplasm outside the wreath) arranged at periphery of collection of histiocytes
- Eosinophils may be present
- Scattered foamy cells may be present

Juvenile xanthogranuloma

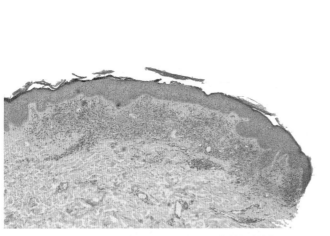
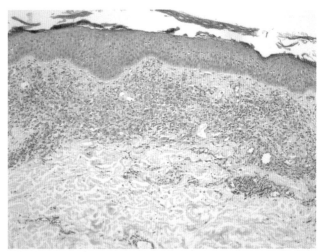
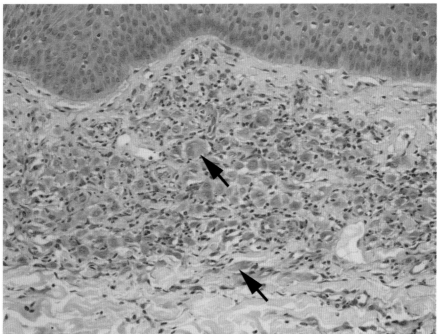

• Oncocytic giant cells (multinucleated cells with ground-glass
  pink cytoplasm) (arrows)

Reticulohistiocytosis

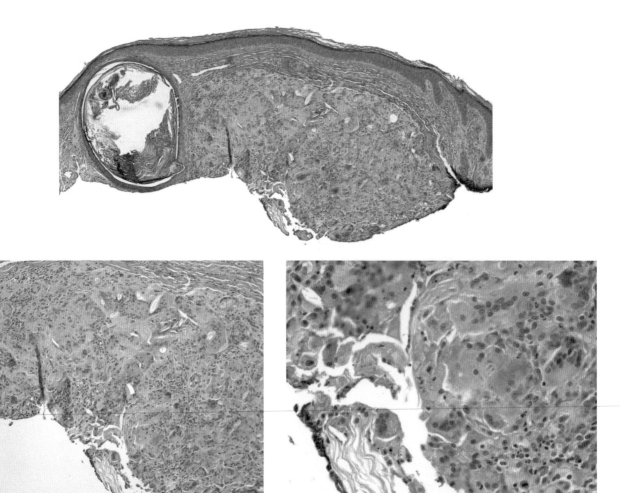

- Foreign-body giant cells (haphazardly arranged nuclei), neutrophils
- Keratin spicules can be seen near/engulfed by multinucleated cells

Ruptured cyst/keratin granuloma

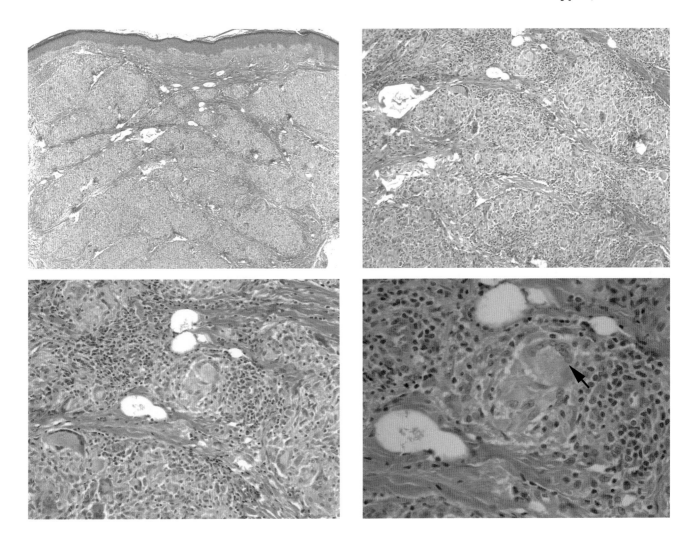

- Langhans giant cells (nuclei arranged in a horseshoe shape) (arrow)
- Epidermis usually normal
- Giant cells within collections of histiocytes that are usually "naked" (lacking surrounding lymphocytes)

Sarcoidosis

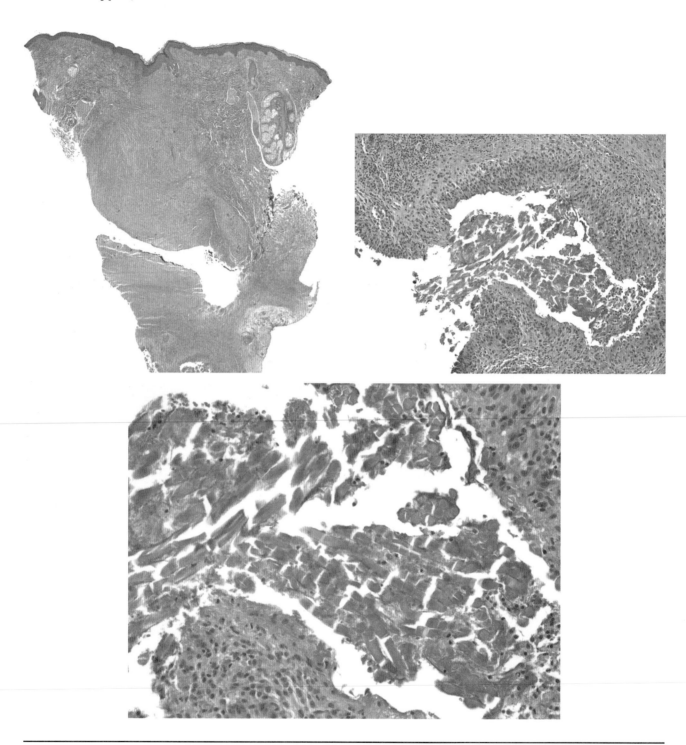

- Foreign-body giant cells
- Cells surrounding suture material (braided in this case)

Suture granuloma

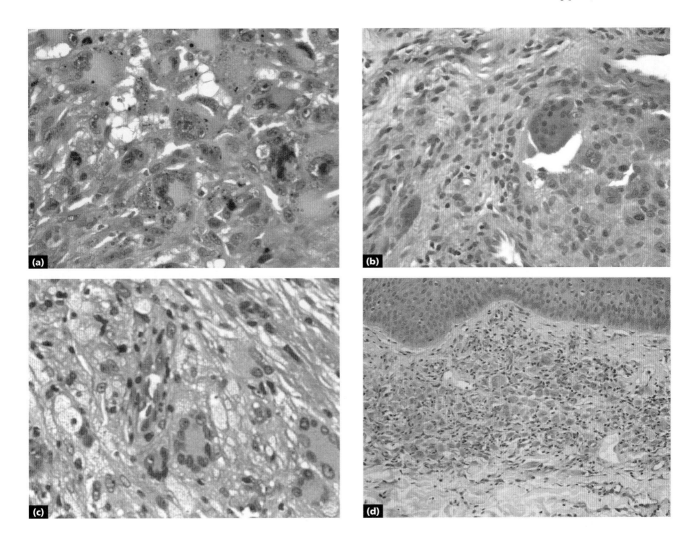

Giant cells

- **a** Atypical fibroxanthoma: atypical nuclei, mitoses
- **b** Giant cell tumor of tendon sheath: osteoclastic giant cells
- **c** Juvenile xanthogranuloma: Touton giant cells
- **d** Reticulohistiocytosis: oncocytic giant cells

Key differences

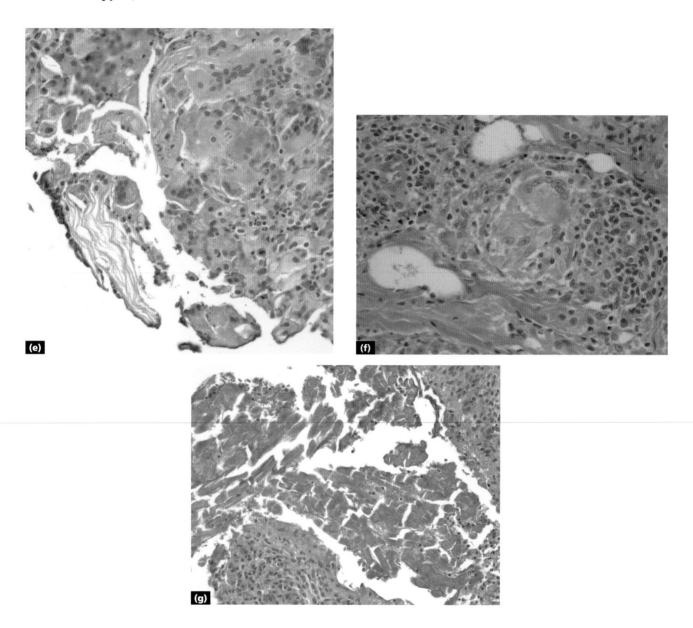

Giant cells (cont.)
- **e** Ruptured cyst/keratin granuloma: foreign-body giant cells, keratin spicules
- **f** Sarcoidosis: Langhans giant cells, naked granulomas
- **g** Suture granuloma: foreign-body giant cells, suture material

- **Note** Infections and scars are other common entities that frequently have giant cells
- **Note** This list is of the classical type of giant cell for each entity; none of the giant cells are pathognomonic

Key differences

4 Color Blue

- Blue tumor, 227
- Blue infiltrate, 235
- Mucin and glands or ducts, 244
- Mucin, 248

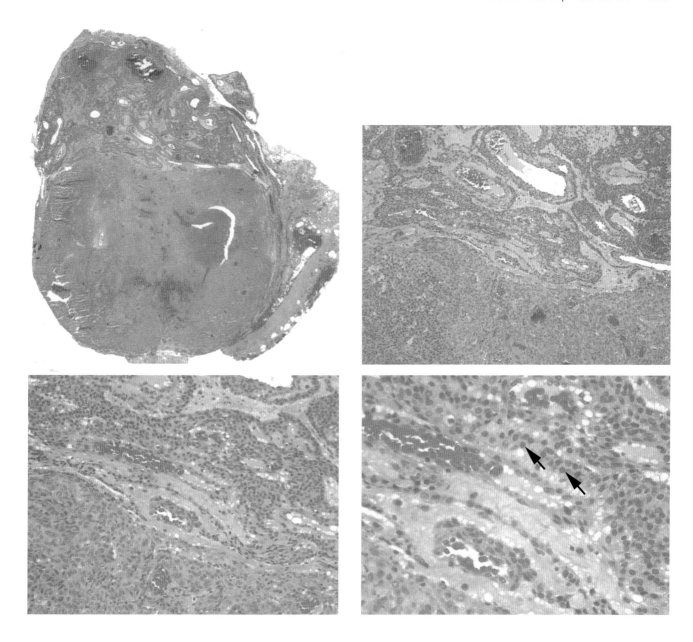

- Blue tumor
- Tumor composed of cells with monomorphous, centrally located, round nuclei (arrows)
- Cells surround vascular spaces

Glomus tumor

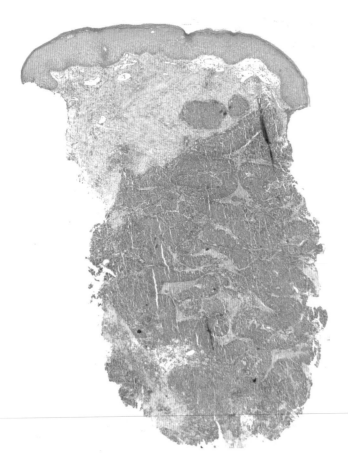
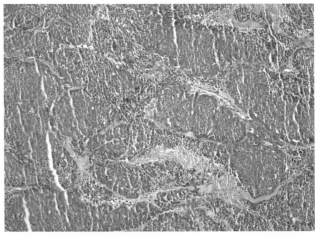
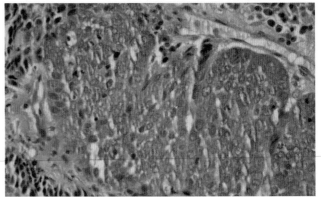

- Blue tumor
- Trabecular or nodular pattern on low power
- Tumor composed of cells with pale nuclei on high power
- Nuclei have a "salt and pepper" look
- Numerous scattered mitoses and necrotic cells

Merkel cell carcinoma

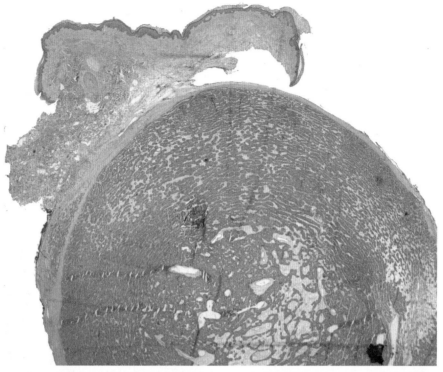

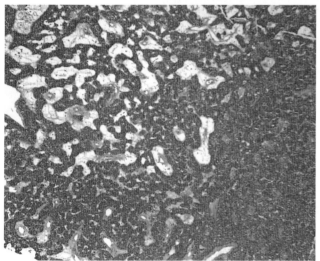 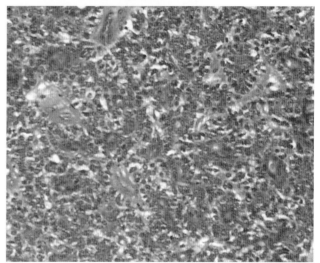

- Blue tumor
- "Blue balls" in the dermis
- Islands of tumor may be peppered by lymphocytes and hyaline pink droplets

- Tumor composed of more peripheral blue cells and more central pale/clear cells that may be arranged in a trabeculated pattern
- Occasional ductal components

Spiradenoma

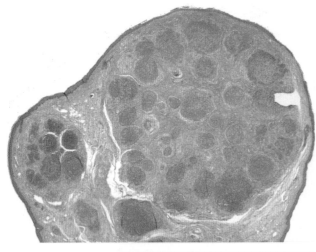
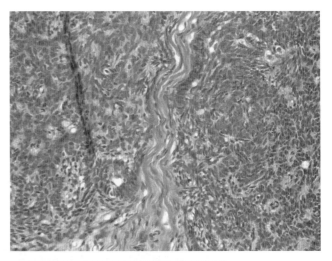
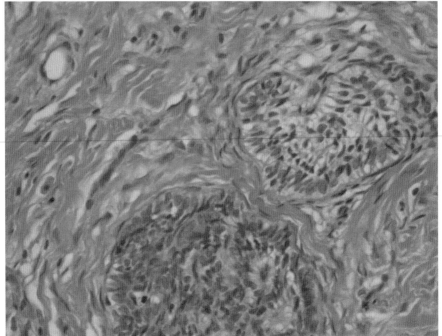

- Blue tumor
- Peripheral palisading
- Generally no epidermal connection

- Well circumscribed with clefts between the tumor as a whole and the normal dermis
- Papillary mesenchymal bodies may be seen

Trichoblastoma

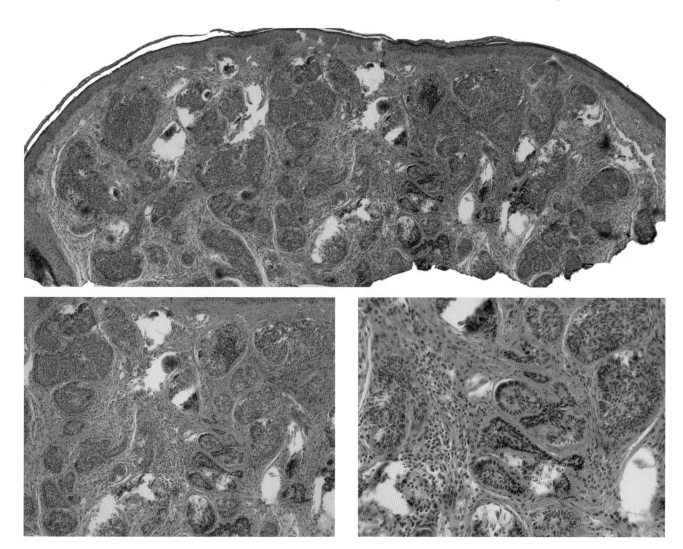

- Blue tumor
- Often an epidermal connection
- Grape-like fronds of cells or reticulated islands of basaloid cells with peripheral palisading
- Fibrotic stroma
- Clefting between the fibrotic stroma and bordering normal dermis
- Papillary mesenchymal bodies may be seen

Trichoepithelioma

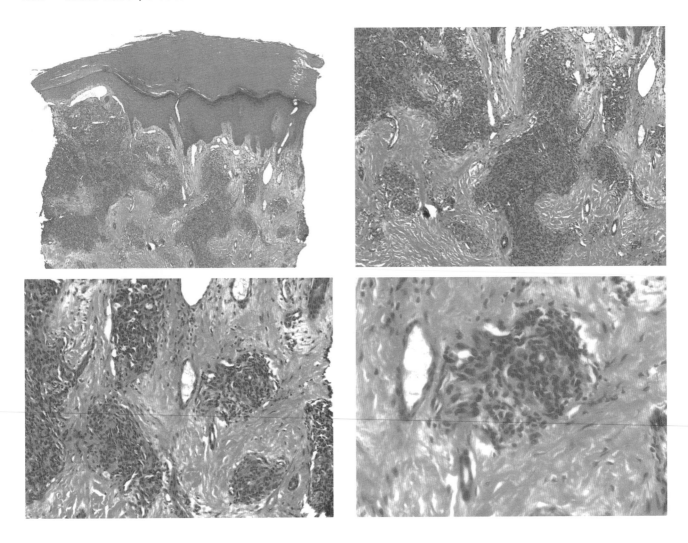

- Blue tumor
- Groups of cells in dermis ("cannon balls") forming small vascular spaces with erythrocytes
- Clefts may be seen around the groups of cells

Tufted hemangioma

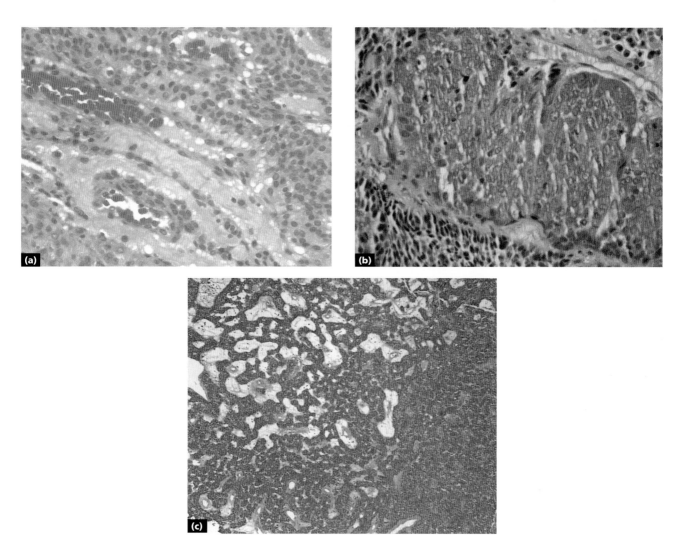

Blue tumors

- **a** Glomus tumor: round monomorphous cells
- **b** Merkel cell carcinoma: pale salt and pepper nuclei
- **c** Spiradenoma: two cell types – pale and blue

Key differences

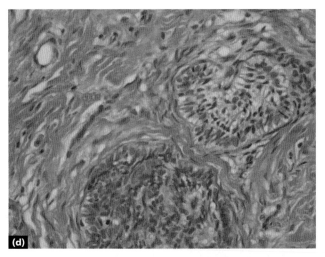

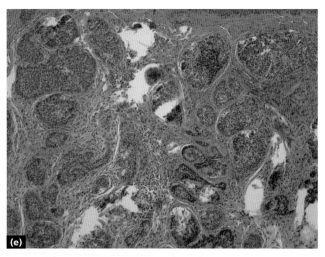

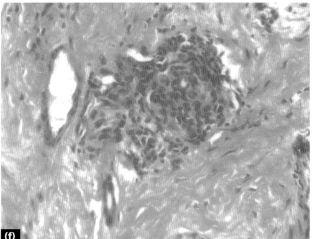

Blue tumors (cont.)

- **d** Trichoblastoma: peripheral palisading, papillary mesenchymal bodies
- **e** Trichoepithelioma: grape-like fronds of cells with peripheral palisading, fibrotic stroma
- **f** Tufted hemangioma: "cannon balls" of blue cells forming vascular spaces
- **Note** Some pathologists consider trichoepithelioma to be a variant of trichoblastoma

Key differences

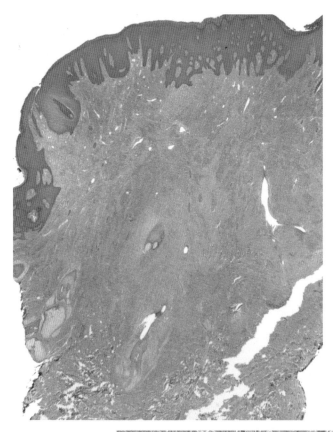
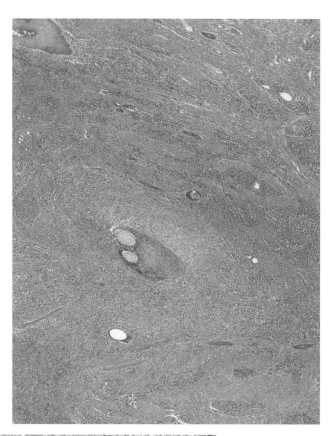
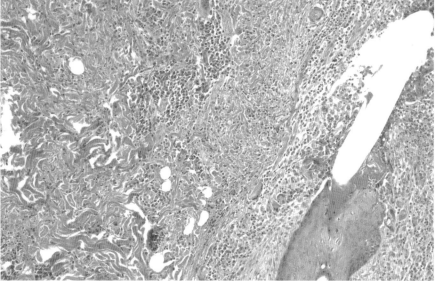

- Blue dense infiltrate
- Lymphoplasmacytic infiltrate surrounds and destroys hair follicles
- Free hair shafts may be seen in the dermis
- Scarring

Acne keloidalis

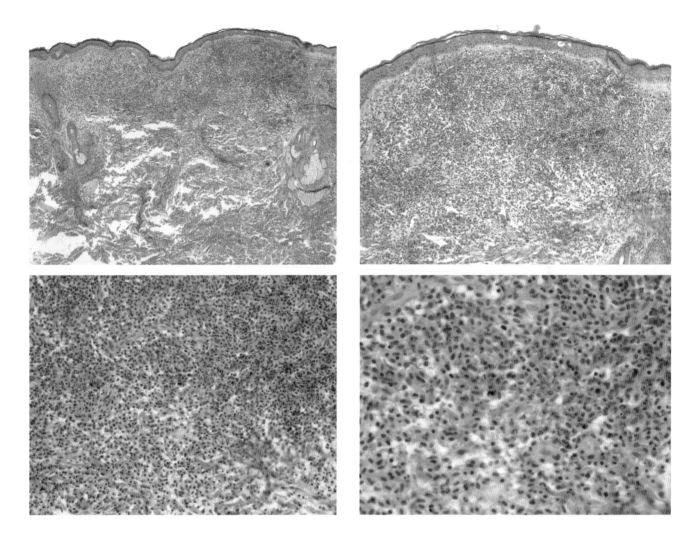

- Blue dense infiltrate
- Grenz zone
- Infiltrate composed of lymphocytes, histiocytes, eosinophils, and neutrophils
- Variable presence of vasculitis

Granuloma faciale

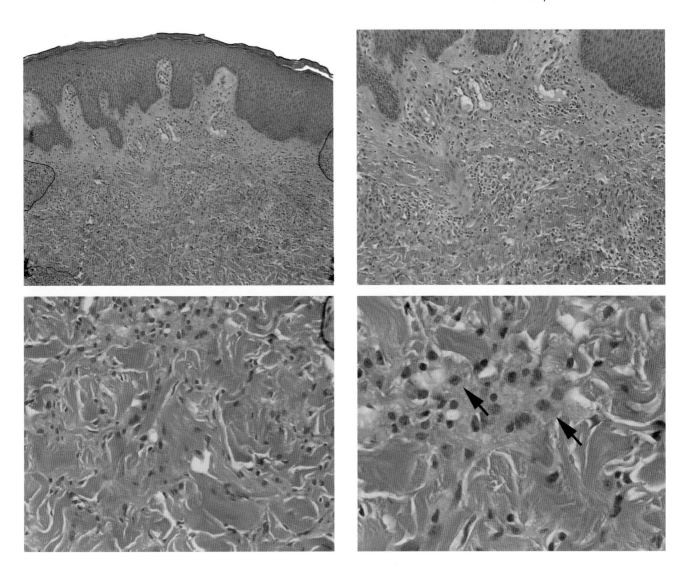

- Blue dense infiltrate
- Infiltrate is perivascular and infiltrating through collagen
- Cells are atypical with slightly granular cytoplasm (arrows)

Leukemia (myelogenous)

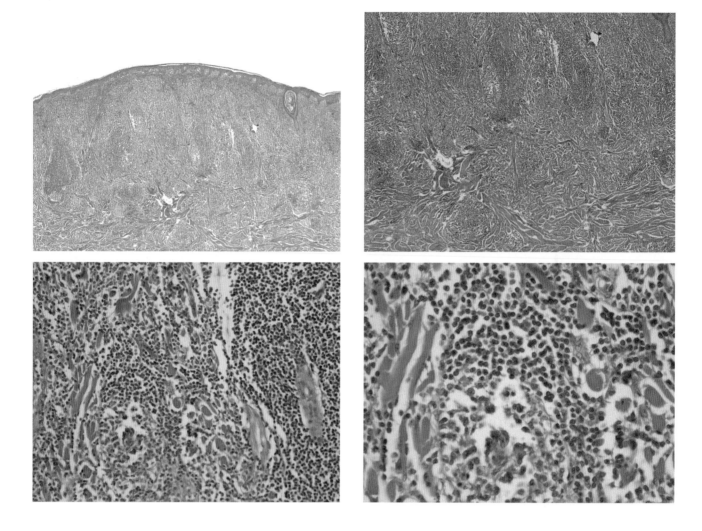

- Blue dense infiltrate
- Infiltrate composed of monomorphous atypical lymphocytes
- Often a "bottom-heavy" infiltrate
- Note that clinical history and special stains may be critical in making the diagnosis

Lymphoma

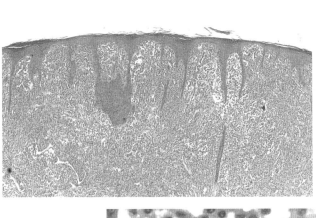
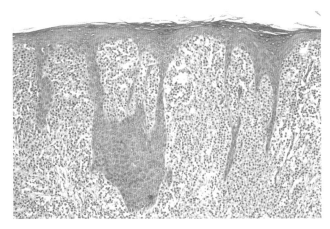
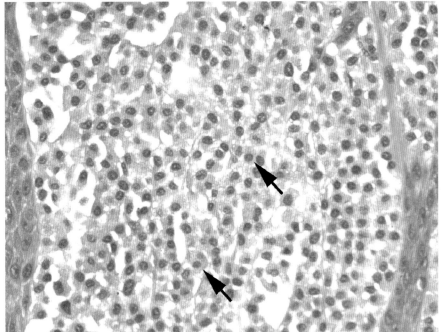

- Blue dense infiltrate
- Infiltrate composed of mast cells (arrows) with "fried egg" appearance (round nucleus, granular cytoplasm)

Mastocytoma

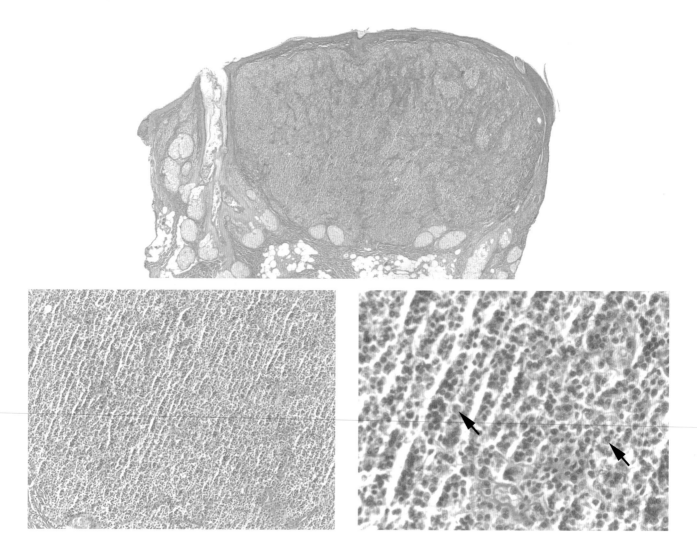

- Blue dense infiltrate
- Infiltrate composed of plasma cells (arrows) with eccentric
  nucleus, perinuclear Hopf (clear space)

Myeloma

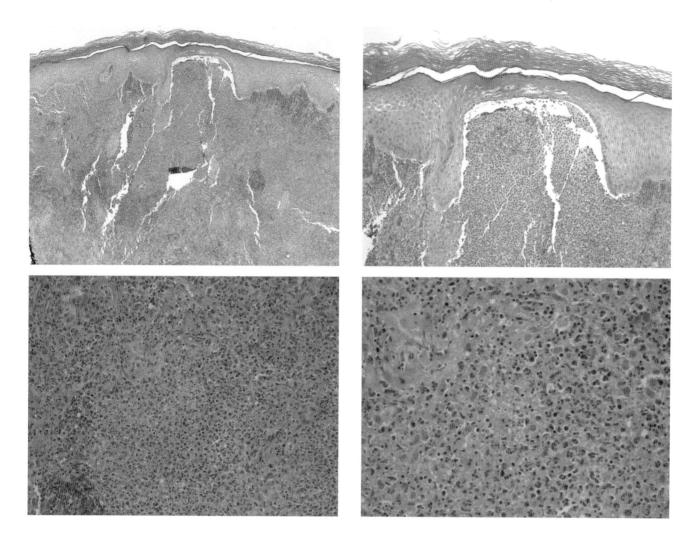

- Blue dense infiltrate
- Papillary dermal edema
- Infiltrate composed of neutrophils
- Generally vasculitis is not prominent

Sweet's syndrome

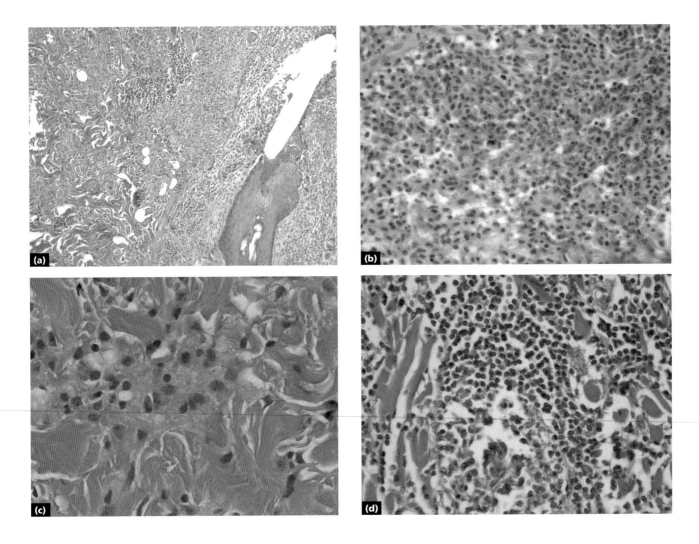

Blue dense infiltrate

- **a** Acne keloidalis: lymphoplasmacytic infiltrate around/destroying hair follicles with scarring
- **b** Granuloma faciale: mixed infiltrate with eosinophils under a grenz zone, vasculitis
- **c** Leukemia (myelogenous): atypical cells with granular cytoplasm around vessels and infiltrating dermis
- **d** Lymphoma: monomorphous lymphocytes filling dermis

Key differences

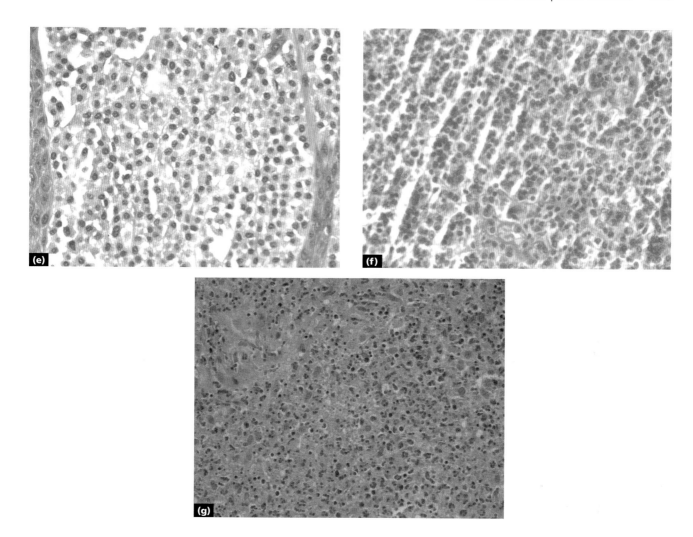

Blue dense infiltrate (cont.)

- **e** Mastocytoma: dense collection of mast cells with "fried egg" appearance
- **f** Myeloma: dense collection of plasma cells
- **g** Sweet's syndrome: infiltrate of neutrophils
- **Note** Infections may also have a dense infiltrate

Key differences

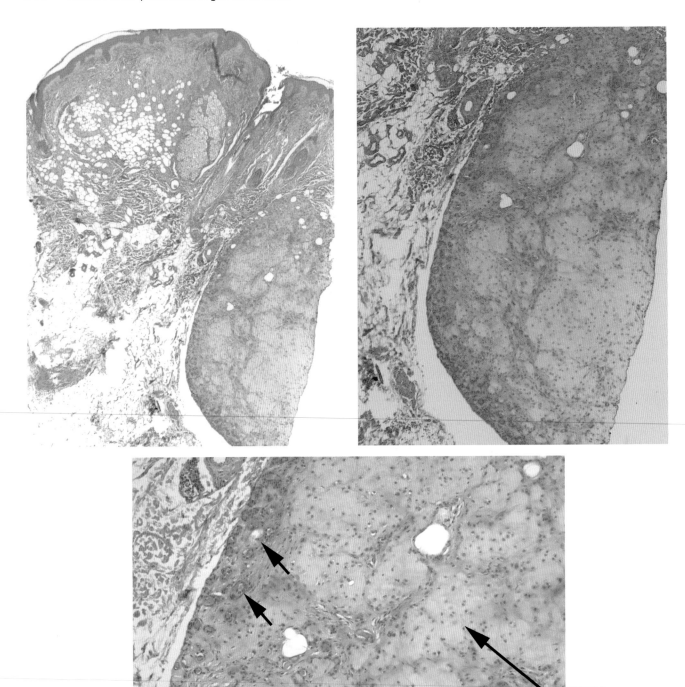

- Mucin and glands or ducts
- Bluish-pink chondroid areas (long arrows) and duct-like spaces (short arrows)
- Well circumscribed

Chondroid syringoma

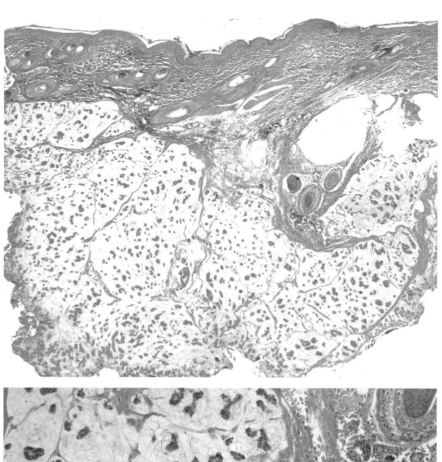

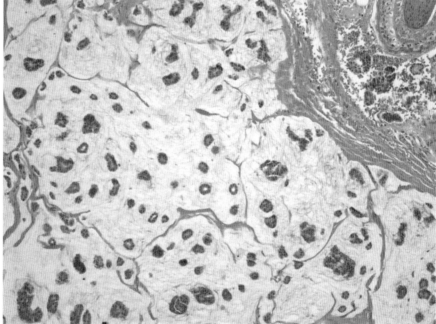

- Mucin and glands or ducts
- Mucin in pools dissecting collagen bundles
- In the center of the pools, there are epithelial islands with variable ductal differentiation

Mucinous carcinoma

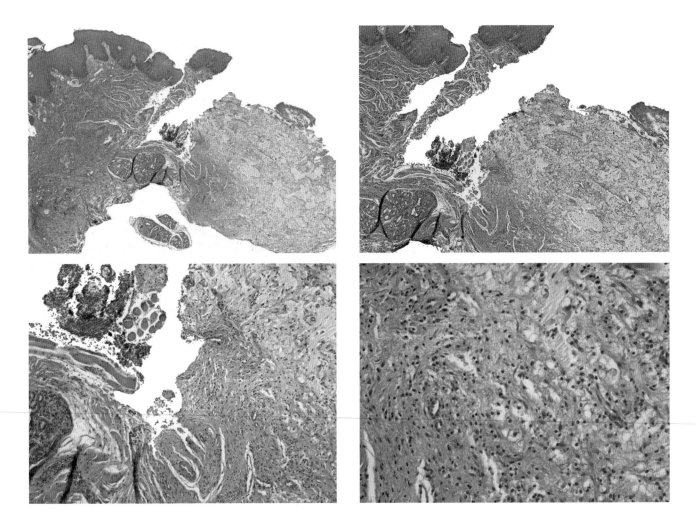

- Mucin and glands or ducts
- Mucin often surrounded by giant cells
- There may be a partial or total epithelial lining
- May see mucosal epithelium and/or minor salivary glands

Mucocele

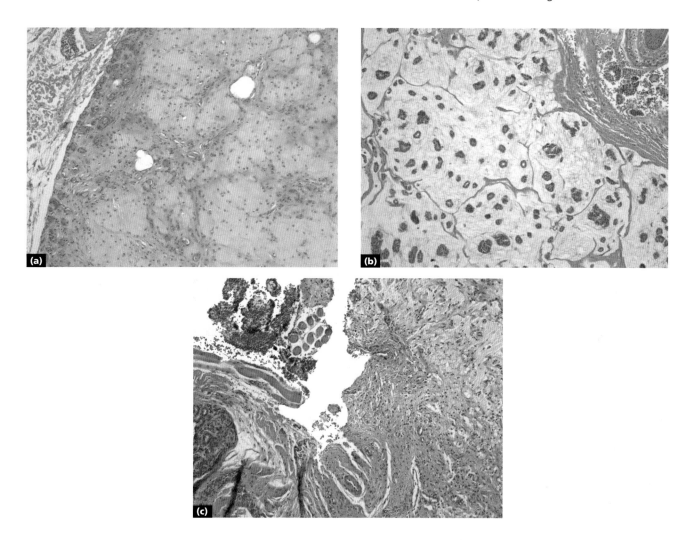

Mucin and glands or ducts

- **a** Chondroid syringoma: well-circumscribed blue–pink cartilaginous area containing duct-like spaces

- **b** Mucinous carcinoma: pools of mucin containing epithelial islands
- **c** Mucocele: pool of mucin with surrounding fibrosis/ inflammation; adjacent salivary glands

Key differences

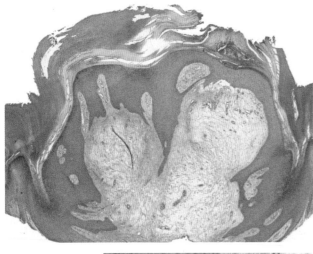
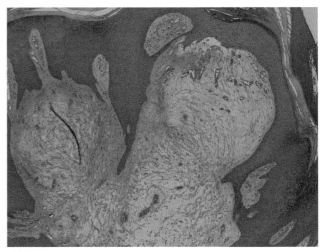
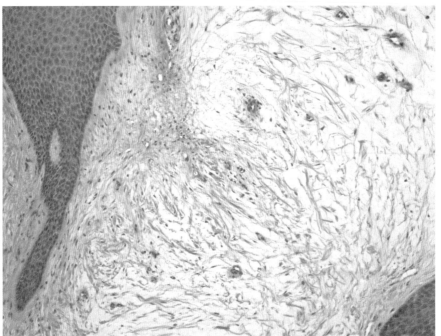

- Well-circumscribed mucin (blue, lacy appearance)
- Acral skin
- Not a true cyst (no epithelial lining)

Digital mucous cyst

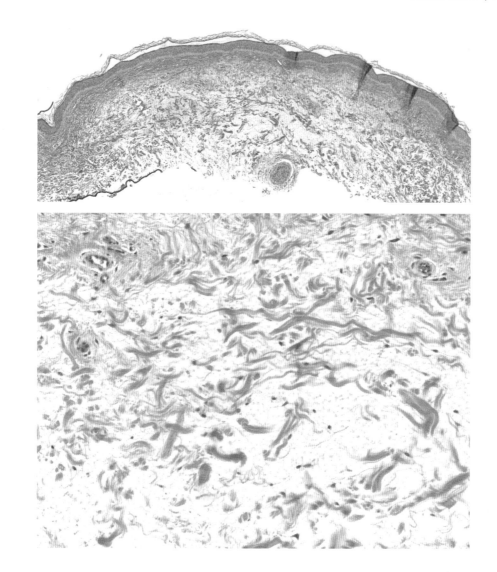

- Well-circumscribed mucin
- Non-acral location

Focal cutaneous mucinosis

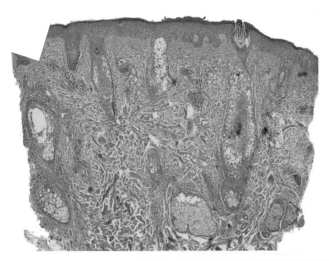
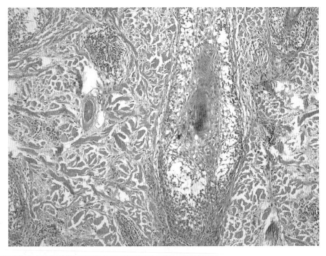
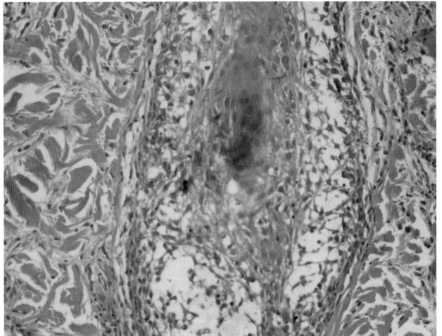

• Mucin within a distorted hair follicle

Follicular mucinosis

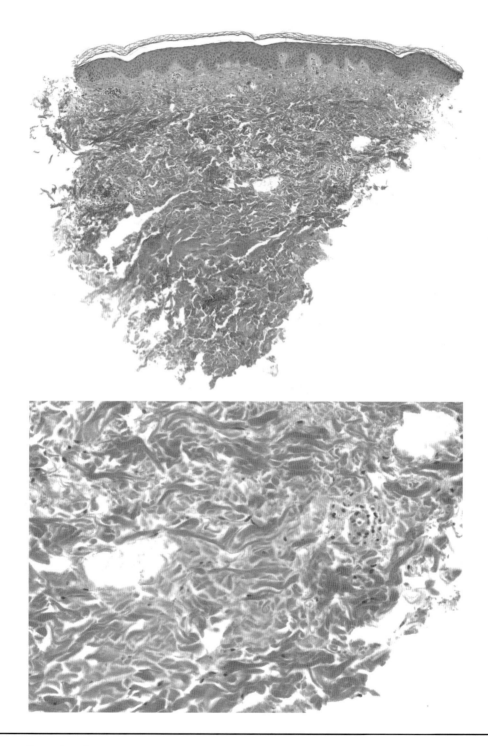

- Mucin between collagen bundles
- Perivascular lymphocytes

Lupus tumidus

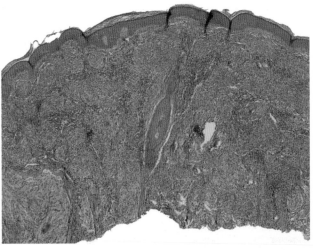
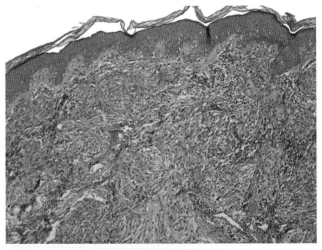
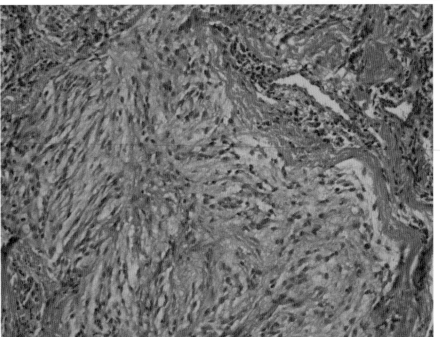

- Variable mucin in nodular collections with spindle cells
- Nodules separated by fibrosis
- Note that lesions with abundant mucin are probably best referred to as nerve sheath myxomas

Neurothekeoma

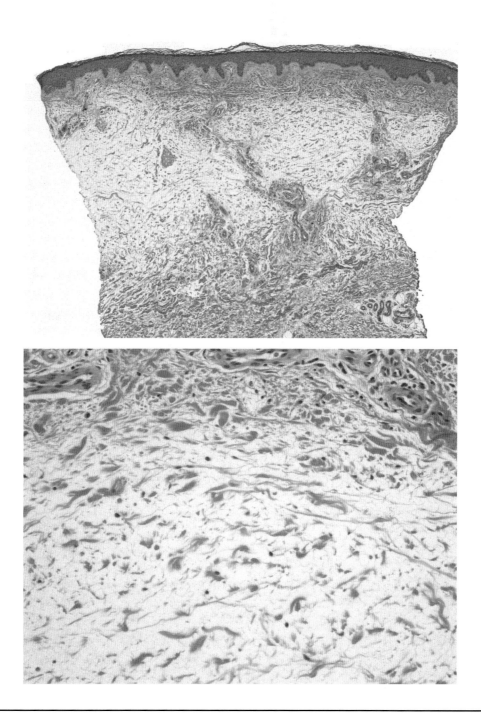

- Mucin filling the dermis (spares papillary dermis)

Pretibial myxedema

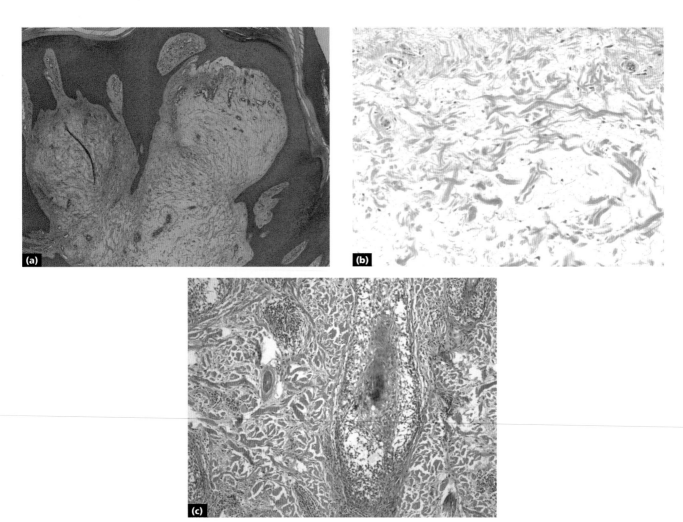

Mucin

- **a** Digital mucous cyst: acral location
- **b** Focal cutaneous mucinosis: non-acral location
- **c** Follicular mucinosis: mucin within follicle

Key differences

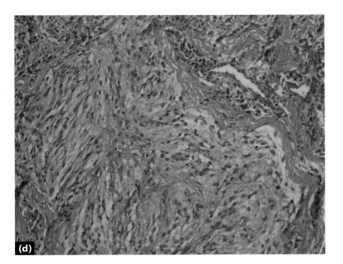

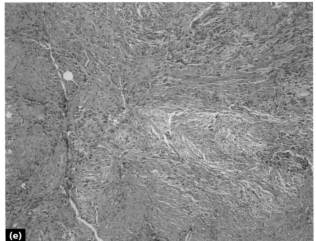

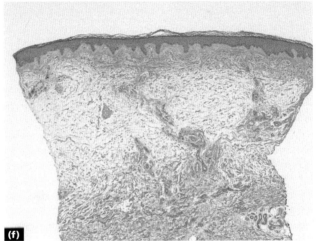

Mucin (cont.)

- **d** Neurothekeoma: lobules of spindle or epithelioid cells in variable myxoid background
- **e** Nodular fasciitis: elongated "tissue culture" cells in myxoid background
- **f** Pretibial myxedema: mucin filling reticular dermis

Key differences

5 **Color Pink**

- Pink material, 259
- Pink dermis, 264
- Epidermal necrosis, 267

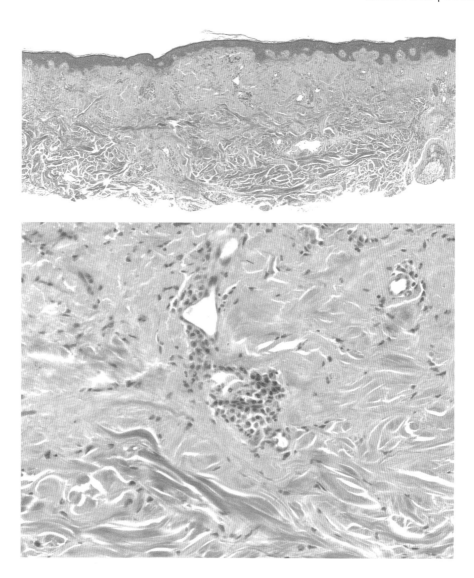

- Amorphous pink material in upper dermis
- Plasma cells

Amyloid

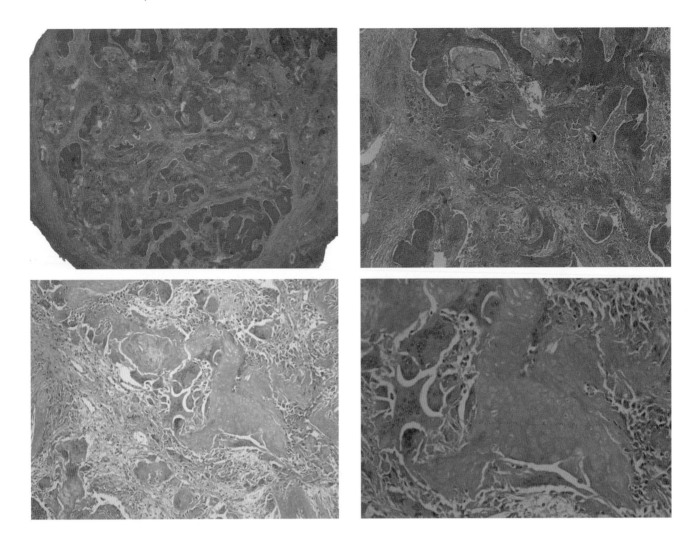

- Pink material with shadows of nuclei within, may have a "butterscotch" color
- Basaloid cells
- Calcification may be present
- Giant cells often seen

Pilomatricoma

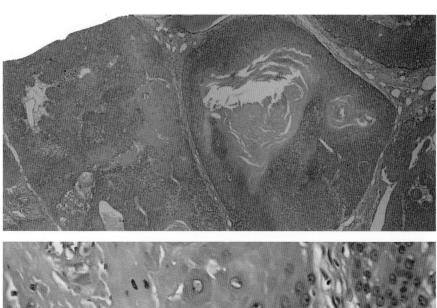

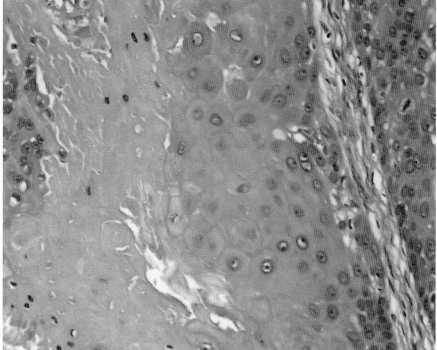

- Pink material that is dense keratin
- Stratified squamous epithelium with no granular layer
  (tricholemmal differentiation)

Proliferating pilar tumor

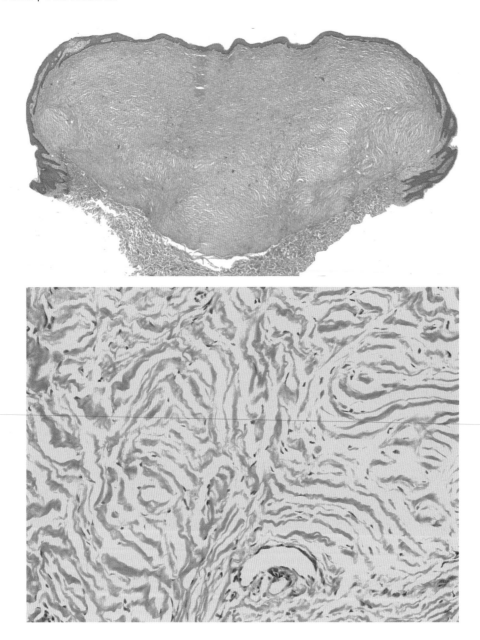

- Pink material arranged in a fenestrated or clefted fashion
- Hyalinized, relatively acellular collagen

Sclerotic fibroma

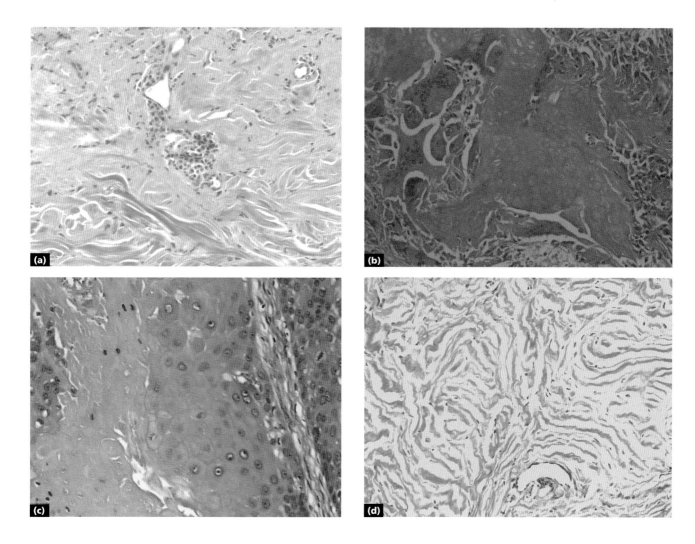

Pink material

- **a** Amyloid: amorphous pink material, plasma cells
- **b** Pilomatricoma: shadow cells, basaloid cells
- **c** Proliferating pilar tumor: dense pink keratin, no granular layer between keratin and epithelium
- **d** Sclerotic fibroma: clefts between strands of sclerotic collagen

Key differences

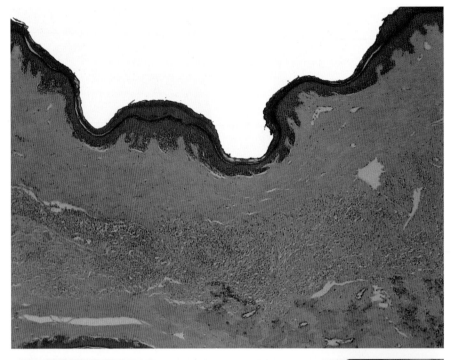

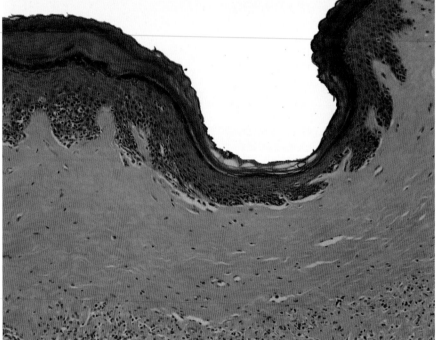

- Pink hyalinized dermis beneath vacuolated basal layer
- Lichenoid infiltrate below hyalinized dermis
- See also p. 89

Lichen sclerosus et atrophicus

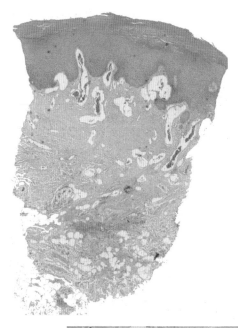
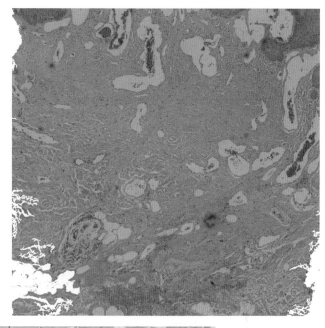
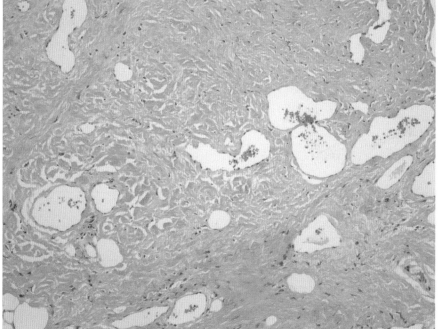

- Pink dermis
- Atypical, bizarre fibroblasts within dermis
- Dilated vessels with plump endothelial cells

Radiation dermatitis

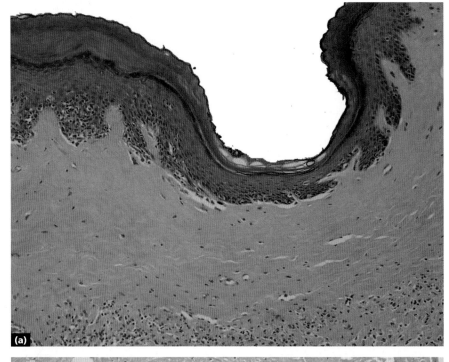

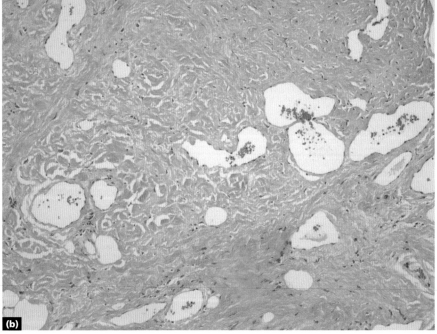

Pink dermis
- **a** Lichen sclerosus et atrophicus: pink band of dermis with inflammation below it (see also p. 93)
- **b** Radiation dermatitis: pink dermis with dilated vessels; atypical fibroblasts on higher power

Key differences

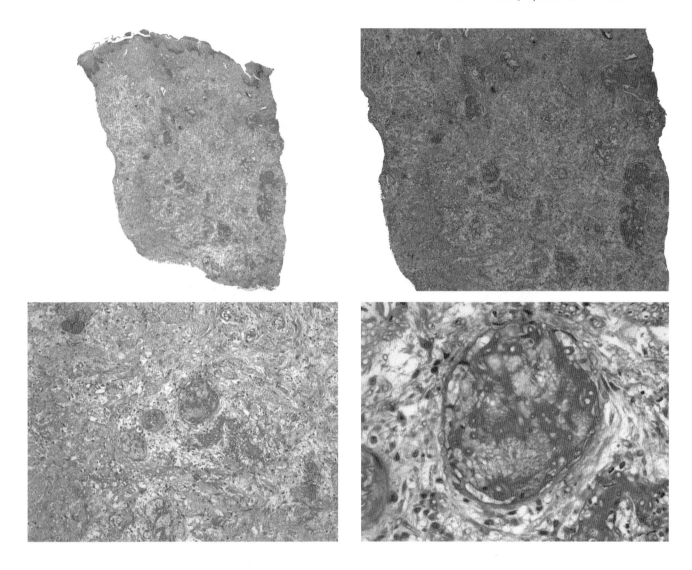

- Epidermal and dermal necrosis
- Vessels necrotic with extravasated erythrocytes and visible fungal hyphae that are septate and branching

Aspergillosis

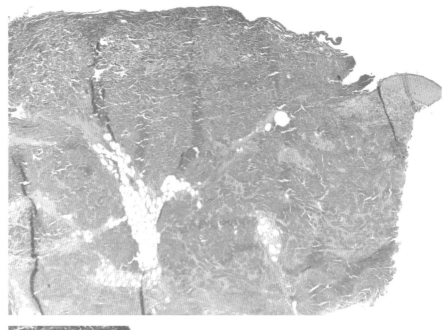

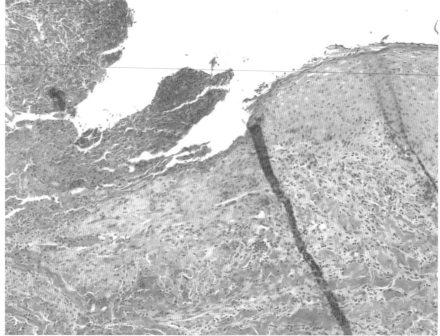

- Epidermal necrosis with variable dermal change
- Reversal of epidermal staining (more basophilic superficially than deep)
- Acute lesions are non-inflammatory

Burn

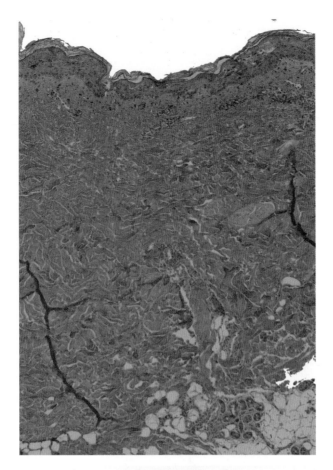

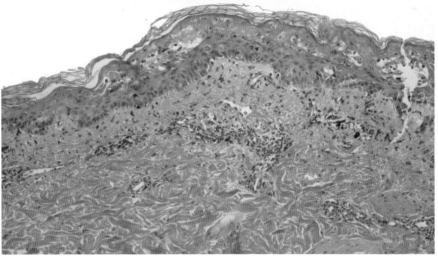

- Epidermal necrosis (linear, primarily affecting basal layer)
  below basket-weave stratum corneum in early lesions

Erythema multiforme

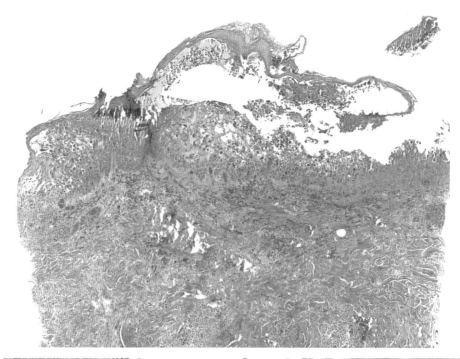

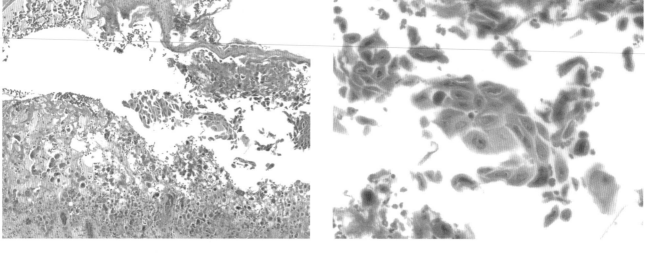

- Epidermal necrosis with acantholytic cells and multinucleated cells
- Follicular necrosis is a clue

Herpes simplex infection

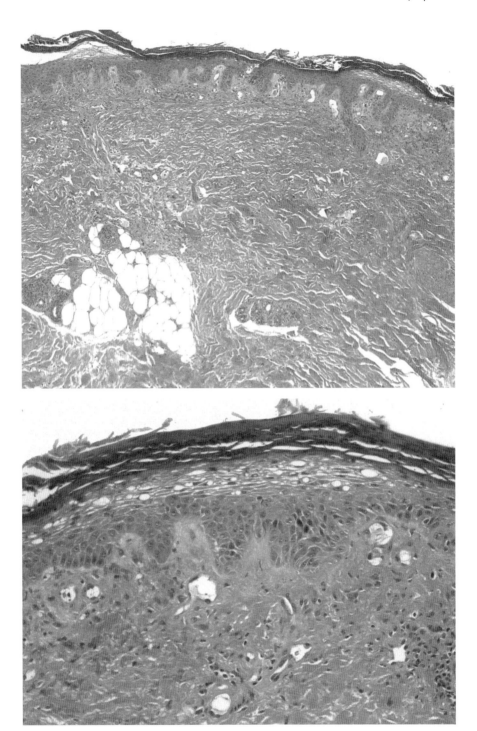

- Epidermal necrosis or pallor underlying parakeratosis
- Basal layer relatively normal

Nutritional deficiency

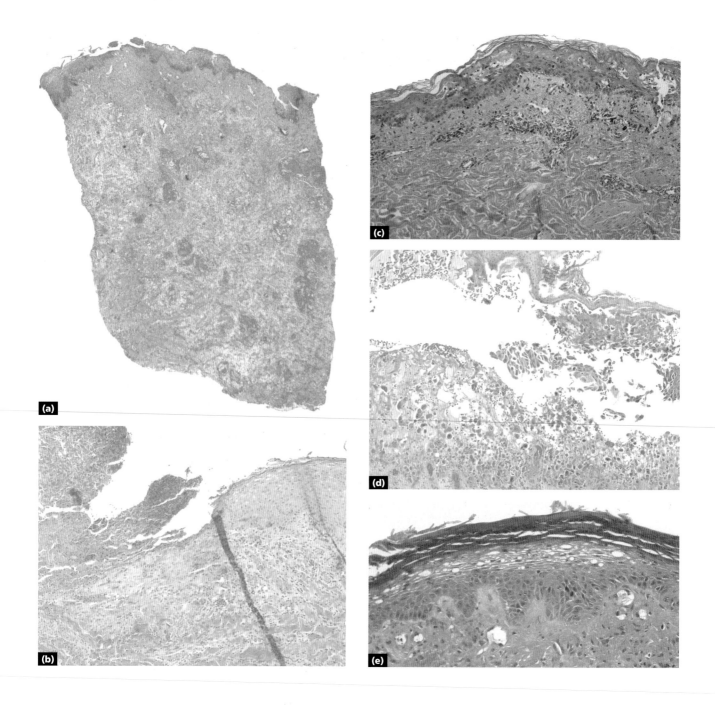

Epidermal necrosis

- **a** Aspergillosis: epidermal and dermal necrosis with fungi in areas of destroyed vessels
- **b** Burn: epidermal necrosis, sharp demarcation
- **c** Erythema multiforme: basket-weave stratum corneum, linear basal cell necrosis
- **d** Herpes simplex infection: acantholysis and multinucleated cells with rimmed chromatin
- **e** Nutritional deficiency: parakeratosis above epidermal necrosis, basal layer often unaffected

Key differences

6 Appendix by Pattern

Polypoid
Accessory digit, 3, 7
Accessory nipple, 4, 7
Accessory tragus, 5, 7
Acquired digital fibrokeratoma, see Digital fibrokeratoma
Digital fibrokeratoma, 6, 7
Fibroepithelial polyp (not pictured)
Fibrous papule, 75, 81
Intradermal nevus (not pictured)
Neurofibroma, 208, 214
Nevus lipomatosus (not pictured)
Umbilical polyp (not pictured)

Square/rectangular
Chronic radiodermatitis, 265
Keloid (not pictured)
Lichen myxedematosus, 12
Morphea, 8, 13
Necrobiosis lipoidica, 9, 13, 39
Nephrogenic systemic fibrosis (not pictured)
Normal back, 10, 13
Scleredema, 11, 14
Scleromyxedema, 12, 14

Regular acanthosis
Bowen's disease, 15, 18
Clear cell acanthoma, 16, 18
Normal elbow (not pictured)
Psoriasis, 17, 18
Inflammatory linear verrucous epidermal
  nevus, 88, 92
Verruciform xanthoma (not pictured)

Pseudoepitheliomatous hyperplasia above abscesses
Atypical mycobacterial infection (not pictured)
Blastomycosis, 19, 22
Chromomycosis, 20, 22
Coccidioidomycosis, 21, 22
Keratoacanthoma (not pictured)
Paracoccidioidomycosis (not pictured)
Pyoderma gangrenosum (not pictured)
Sporotrichosis (not pictured)

Tuberculosis verrucosa cutis (not pictured)
Halogenoderma/bromoderma (not pictured)

Proliferation downward from epidermis
Fibroepithelioma of Pinkus, 23, 30
Fibrofolliculoma, 24, 30
Inverted follicular keratosis, 25, 30
Nevus sebaceous of Jadassohn, 26, 30
Poroma, 27, 31
Sebaceus adenoma, 186, 192
Seborrheic keratosis, reticulated (not pictured)
Syringofibroadenoma (not pictured)
Trichilemmoma, 28, 31
Tumor of the follicular infundibulum, 29, 31

Central pore
Dilated pore of Winer, 32, 35
Pilar sheath acanthoma, 33, 35
Trichofolliculoma, 34, 35
Sebaceous hyperplasia (not pictured)

Palisading reactions
Churg–Strauss (not pictured)
Gout, 36, 39
Granuloma annulare, 37, 39
Interstitial granulomatous dermatitis (not pictured)
Rheumatoid nodule, 38, 39
Necrobiosis lipoidica, 9, 13, 39
Wegener's granulomatosis (not pictured)

Space with a lining
Angiokeratoma, 124, 130
Apocrine hidrocystoma, 40, 49
Auricular pseudocyst, 41, 49
Branchial cleft cyst, 42, 49
Bronchogenic cyst (not pictured)
Cutaneous ciliated cyst, 43, 50
Cutaneous endometriosis, 44, 50
Dermoid cyst, 45, 50
Epidermal inclusion cyst, 46, 51
Lymphangioma, 127, 131
Median raphe cyst (not pictured)
Pilar cyst, 47, 51

Steatocystoma, 48, 51
Thyroglossal duct cyst (not pictured)
Venous lake (not pictured)
Glomangioma (not pictured)

Cords and tubules
Desmoplastic trichoepithelioma, 52, 57
Metastatic breast carcinoma, 53, 57
Microcystic adnexal carcinoma, 54, 57
Morpheaform basal cell carcinoma, 55, 58
Syringoma, 56, 58

Papillated dermal tumor
Aggressive digital papillary adenocarcinoma, 59, 64
Hidradenoma papilliferum, 60, 64
Papillary eccrine adenoma, 61, 64
Syringocystadenoma papilliferum, 62, 65
Tubular apocrine adenoma, 63, 65

Circular dermal islands
Adenoid cystic carcinoma, 66, 69
Cylindroma, 67, 69
Spiradenoma, 229, 233
Trichoadenoma, 68, 69
Trichoblastoma, 230, 234

(Suggestion of) vessels
Angioleiomyoma, 70, 80
Angiolymphoid hyperplasia with eosinophilia, 71, 80
Angiosarcoma, 72, 80
Bacillary angiomatosis, 73, 74, 81
Chondrodermatitis nodularis helicis, 85, 92
Fibrous papule, 75, 81
Glomus tumor/glomangioma, 227, 233
Kaposi's sarcoma, 76, 81
Pyogenic granuloma, 77, 82
Stasis dermatitis, 78, 82
Targetoid hemangioma, 79, 82

Hyperkeratosis
Chondrodermatitis nodularis helicis, 85, 92
Dermatophytosis, 95, 96
Discoid lupus erythematosus, 86, 92
Epidermolytic hyperkeratosis, 99, 105
Flegel's disease, 87, 92
Ichthyosis vulgaris (not pictured)
Inflammatory linear verrucous epidermal nevus, 88, 92
Lichen planus, 144, 148
Lichen sclerosus et atrophicus, 89, 93, 264, 266
Pityriasis rubra pilaris, 90, 93
Porokeratosis, 91, 93

Parakeratosis
Axillary granular parakeratosis, 94, 96
Bowen's disease, 15, 18

Dermatophytosis, 95, 96
Nutritional deficiency, 271, 272
Papulosquamous diseases (not all are pictured), 17 ,18, 90, 93
Pityriasis lichenoides et varioliformis acuta, 146, 148
Porokeratosis, 91, 93
Spongiotic diseases (not all are pictured), 78, 82, 117, 118, 135, 136
Tinea versicolor (not pictured)

Upper epidermal change
Bowen's disease, 15, 18
Clonal seborrheic keratosis, 97, 105
Epidermodysplasia verruciformis, 98, 105
Epidermolytic hyperkeratosis, 99, 105
Myrmecium, 100, 105
Orf, 101, 106
Paget's disease, 102, 106
Verruca plana, 103, 106
Verruca vulgaris, 104, 106

Acantholysis
Acantholytic acanthoma (not pictured)
Actinic keratosis (not pictured)
Acantholytic dyskeratotic acanthoma (not pictured)
Darier's disease, 107, 115
Grover's disease, 108, 115
Hailey–Hailey disease, 109, 115
Herpes virus infection, 110, 115
Pemphigus foliaceus, 111, 116
Pemphigus vulgaris, 112, 116
Pityriasis rubra pilaris, 90, 93
Squamous cell carcinoma, 113, 116
Warty dyskeratoma, 114, 116

Eosinophilic spongiosis
Allergic contact dermatitis, 117, 122
Arthropod bite reaction, 118, 122
Bullous pemphigoid, 122, 125, 130
Incontinentia pigmenti, 119, 123
Pemphigoid gestationis, 125
Pemphigus vegetans, 120, 123
Pemphigus vulgaris, 112, 116
Scabies, 121, 123

Subepidermal space cleft
Angiokeratoma, 124, 130
Bullous pemphigoid, 122, 125, 130
Dermatitis herpetiformis, 126, 130
Diabetic bullae (not pictured)
Epidermolysis bullosa (not pictured)
Erythema multiforme, 269, 272
Herpes gestationis, 125
Lichen planus (not pictured)

Lymphangioma, 127, 131
Phototoxic reactions (not pictured)
Polymorphous light eruption, 128, 131
Porphyria cutanea tarda, 129, 131
Pseudoporphyria (not pictured)
Suction blister (not pictured)
Sweet's syndrome, 241, 243

Perivascular infiltrate
Erythema annulare centrifuguum (not pictured)
Guttate psoriasis (not pictured)
Gyrate erythema, 132, 136
Leukocytoclastic vasculitis, 133, 136
Lymphocytic angiitis (not pictured)
Pigmented purpuric dermatosis, 134, 136
Pityriasis rosea, 135, 136

Band-like upper dermal infiltrate
Fixed drug reaction, 141, 147
Langerhans cell histiocytosis, 137, 140
Lichen planus, 144, 148
Mastocytosis, 138, 140
Mycosis fungoides, 139, 140

Interface reaction
Benign lichenoid keratosis (not pictured)
Discoid lupus erythematosus, 86, 92
Erythema multiforme, 269, 272
Fixed drug reaction, 141, 147
Graft-versus-host disease, 142, 147
Halo nevus (not pictured)
Lichen nitidus, 143, 147
Lichen planus, 144, 148
Lichen sclerosus et atrophicus, 89, 93, 264, 266
Lichen striatus, 145, 148
Pigmented purpuric dermatosis, 134, 136
Pityriasis lichenoides et varioliformis acuta, 146, 148
Porokeratosis, 91, 93
Regressed melanoma (not pictured)
Secondary syphilis (not pictured)
Some neoplasms (not pictured)

Dermal material
Amyloidosis, nodular, 149, 159
Calcinosis cutis, 150, 159
Erythropoietic protoporphyria, 151, 159
Gel foam, 152, 159
Gout, 36, 39
Lipoid proteinosis, 153, 160
Ochronosis, 154, 160
Osteoma cutis, 155, 160
Paraffinoma, 156, 161
Pseudoxanthoma elasticum, 157, 161
Tattoo, 158, 161
See also **Mucin**, 248 and **Pink material**, 259

Change in the fat
Angiolipoma, 162, 171
Dermatofibrosarcoma protuberans (often extends into the fat), 205, 213
Erythema induratum, 163, 171
Erythema nodosum, 164, 171
Hibernoma, 179, 190
Lipodermatosclerosis, 165, 172
Lupus profundus, 166, 172
Nodular fasciitis (often deep in the fat), 209, 214, 255
Other adipose tumors (not pictured)
Other panniculitides (not pictured)
Pancreatic fat necrosis, 167, 172
Polyarteritis nodosa, 168, 173
Post-steroid panniculitis, 169
Sclerema neonatorum (not pictured)
Subcutaneous fat necrosis of the newborn, 169, 173
Subcutaneous T-cell lymphoma, 170, 173

"Clear cells"
Clear cell acanthoma, 16, 18
Cryptococcosis, gelatinous, 177, 190
Granular cell tumor, 178, 190
Hibernoma, 179, 190
Leishmaniasis, 180, 190
Lepromatous leprosy, 181, 191
Lipoma, 182, 191
Melanoma, balloon cell, 183, 191
Nodular hidradenoma, 184, 192
Other clear cell neoplasms (e.g. clear cell basal cell carcinoma) (not pictured)
Renal cell carcinoma, 185, 192
Sebaceous adenoma, 186, 192
Trichilemmoma, 28, 31
Xanthelasma, 187, 193
Xanthogranuloma, 188, 193
Xanthoma, 189, 193

Melanocytic cells
Blue nevus, 194, 201
Blue nevus, cellular, 203, 213
Deep penetrating nevus, 195, 201
Melanoma, 196, 201
Melanoma, desmoplastic, 197, 201
Other melanocytic tumors/proliferations (not pictured)
Pigmented spindle cell nevus of Reed, 198, 202
Recurrent nevus, 199, 202
Spitz nevus, 200, 202

Spindle cells
Atypical fibroxanthoma, 216, 223
Blue nevus, cellular, 203, 213
Dermatofibroma, 204, 213
Dermatofibrosarcoma protuberans, 205, 213
Fibrous papule, 75, 81

Infantile digital fibromatosis, 206, 213
Kaposi's sarcoma, 76, 81
Leiomyoma, 207, 214
Neurofibroma, 208, 214
Neurothekeoma, 252, 255
Nodular fasciitis, 209, 214, 255
Other fibrous tumors (not pictured)
Other neural tumors (not pictured)
Other smooth muscle tumors (not pictured)
Palisaded encapsulated neuroma, 210, 215
Scar, 211, 215
Schwannoma, 212, 215
Squamous cell carcinoma, 113, 116

Giant cells
Atypical fibroxanthoma, 216, 223
Erythema nodosum, 164, 171
Giant cell tumor of tendon sheath, 217, 223
Infections (not pictured)
Juvenile xanthogranuloma, 218, 223
Mucocele, 246, 247
Necrobiosis lipoidica, 9, 13, 39
Pilomatricoma, 260
Reticulohistiocytosis, 219, 223
Ruptured cyst/keratin granuloma, 220, 224
Sarcoidosis, 221, 224
Scar (not pictured)
Suture granuloma, 222, 224

Blue tumor
Basal cell carcinoma, morpheaform, 55, 58
Glomus tumor, 227, 233
Lymphoma, 238, 242
Merkel cell carcinoma, 228, 233
Sebaceoma (not pictured)
Spiradenoma, 229, 233
Trichoblastoma, 230, 234
Trichoepithelioma, 231, 234
Tufted hemangioma, 232, 234

Blue dense infiltrate
Acne keloidalis, 235, 242
Granuloma faciale, 236, 242
Infections (not pictured)
Leukemia (myelogenous), 237, 242
Lymphoma, 238, 242
Mastocytoma, 239, 243
Myeloma, 240, 243
Sweet's syndrome, 241, 243

Mucin and glands or ducts
Chondroid syringoma, 244, 247
Mucinous carcinoma, 245, 247
Mucocele, 246, 247

Mucin
Digital mucous cyst, 248, 254
Focal cutaneous mucinosis, 249, 254
Follicular mucinosis, 250, 254
Lichen myxedematosus, 12
Lupus tumidus, 251
Neurothekeoma, 252, 255
Nodular fasciitis, 209, 214, 255
Pretibial myxedema, 253, 255
Reticular erythematous mucinosis (not pictured)
Scleredema, 11, 14
Scleromyxedema, 12, 14

Pink material
Amyloid, 259, 263
Colloid milium (not pictured)
Erythropoietic protoporphyria, 151, 159
Gout, 36, 39
Lichen sclerosus et atrophicus, 89, 93, 264, 266
Lipoid proteinosis, 153, 160
Pilar cyst, 47, 51
Pilomatricoma, 260, 263
Proliferating pilar tumor, 261, 263
Rheumatoid nodule, 38, 39
Sclerotic fibroma, 262, 263

Pink dermis
Lichen sclerosus et atrophicus, 89, 93, 264, 266
Morphea, 8, 13
Radiation dermatitis, 265, 266

Epidermal necrosis
Aspergillosis, 267, 272
Burn, 268, 272
Erythema multiforme, 269, 272
Herpes simplex infection, 270, 272
Nutritional deficiency, 271, 272
Pressure necrolysis (not pictured)

"Normal" skin on low power
Anetoderma (not pictured)
Connective tissue nevus (not pictured)
Dermatophyte/tinea versicolor* (not pictured)
Erythema dyschromicum perstans* (not pictured)
Ichthyosis vulgaris (not pictured)
Scleredema, 11, 14
Vitiligo (not pictured)
Macular amyloidosis* (not pictured)
Urticaria (not pictured)
Telangiectasia macularis eruptiva perstans (TMEP) (not pictured)
Argyria (not pictured)

*When subtle

7 Index by Histological Category

Acantholytic disorders
Darier's disease, 107, 115
Grover's disease, 108, 115
Hailey–Hailey disease, 109, 115
Herpes virus infection, 110, 115
Pemphigus foliaceus, 111, 116
Pemphigus vegetans, 120, 123
Pemphigus vulgaris, 112, 116
Squamous cell carcinoma, acantholytic, 113, 116
Warty dyskeratoma, 114, 116

Benign tumors
Adipose tumors
Angiolipoma, 162, 171
Hibernoma, 179, 190
Lipoma, 182, 191

Adnexal tumors
Follicular
Desmoplastic trichoepithelioma, 52, 57
Fibroepithelioma of Pinkus, 23, 30
Fibrofolliculoma, 24, 30
Pilar sheath acanthoma, 33, 35
Pilomatricoma, 260, 263
Trichilemmoma, 28, 31
Trichoadenoma, 68, 69
Trichoblastoma, 230, 234
Trichoepithelioma, 231, 234
Trichofolliculoma, 34, 35
Tumor of the follicular infundibulum, 29, 31

Glandular (apocrine and eccrine)
Apocrine hidrocystoma, 40, 49
Chondroid syringoma, 244, 247
Cylindroma, 67, 69
Hidradenoma papilliferum, 60, 64
Nodular hidradenoma, 184, 192
Papillary eccrine adenoma, 61, 64
Poroma, 27, 31
Spiradenoma, 229, 233
Syringocystadenoma papilliferum, 62, 65
Syringoma, 56, 58
Tubular apocrine adenoma, 63, 65

Sebaceous
Nevus sebaceus of Jadassohn, 26, 30
Sebaceous adenoma, 186, 192

Fibrous tumors
Dermatofibroma, 204, 213
Dermatofibrosarcoma protuberans, 205, 213
Digital fibrokeratoma, 6, 7
Fibrous papule, 75, 81
Giant cell tumor of tendon sheath, 217, 223
Infantile digital fibromatosis, 206, 213
Nodular fasciitis, 209, 214, 255
Scar, 211, 215
Sclerotic fibroma, 262, 263

Melanocytic tumors
Blue nevus, 194, 201
Blue nevus, cellular, 203, 213
Deep penetrating nevus, 195, 201
Pigmented spindle cell nevus of Reed, 198, 202
Recurrent nevus, 199, 202
Spitz nevus, 200, 202

Miscellaneous tumors
Bronchogenic cyst, 51
Clear cell acanthoma, 16, 18
Cutaneous ciliated cyst, 43, 50
Dilated pore of Winer, 32, 35
Epidermal inclusion cyst, 46, 51
Granular cell tumor, 178, 190
Inverted follicular keratosis, 25, 30
Mastocytoma, 239, 243
Pilar cyst, 47, 51
Seborrheic keratosis, clonal type, 97, 105
Steatocystoma, 48, 51

Neural tumors
Accessory digit, 3, 7
Palisaded encapsulated neuroma, 210, 215
Neurofibroma, 208, 214
Neurothekeoma, 252, 255
Schwannoma, 212, 215

Smooth muscle tumors
Accessory nipple, 4, 7
Angioleiomyoma, 70, 80
Leiomyoma, 207, 214

Vascular tumors
Angiokeratoma, 124, 130
Angiolymphoid hyperplasia with eosinophilia, 71, 80
Glomus tumor, 227, 233
Lymphangioma, 127, 131
Pyogenic granuloma, 77, 82
Targetoid hemangioma, 79, 82
Tufted hemangioma, 232, 234

Connective tissue disorders
Discoid lupus erythematosus, 86, 92
Lichen sclerosus et atrophicus, 89, 93, 264, 266
Lupus profundus, 166, 172
Lupus tumidus, 251
Morphea, 8, 13
Polyarteritis nodosa, 168, 173
Rheumatoid nodule, 38, 39
Scleredema, 11, 14
Scleromyxedema, 12, 14

Depositions
Endogenous material
Amyloidosis, 149, 159, 259
Calcinosis cutis, 150, 159
Digital mucous cyst, 248, 254
Erythropoietic protoporphyria, 151, 159
Focal cutaneous mucinosis, 249, 254
Follicular mucinosis, 250, 254
Gout, 36, 39
Lipoid proteinosis, 153, 160
Mucocele, 246, 247
Osteoma cutis, 155, 160
Pretibial myxedema, 253, 255
Pseudoxanthoma elasticum, 157, 161

Foreign material
Gel foam, 152, 159
Ochronosis, 154, 160
Paraffinoma, 156, 161
Tattoo, 158, 161

Genodermatoses
Epidermolytic hyperkeratosis, 99, 105
Erythropoietic protoporphyria, 151, 159
Incontinentia pigmenti, 119, 123
Lipoid proteinosis, 153, 160

Granulomatous
Granuloma annulare, 37, 39

Necrobiosis lipoidica, 9, 13, 39
Rheumatoid nodule, 38, 39
Ruptured cyst/keratin granuloma, 220, 224
Sarcoidosis, 221, 224
Suture granuloma, 222, 224

Histiocytic
Langerhans cell histiocytosis, 137, 140
Reticulohistiocytosis, 219, 223
Xanthelasma, 187, 193
Xanthogranuloma, 188, 193, 218, 223
Xanthoma, 189, 193

Infections
Aspergillosis, 267, 272
Bacillary angiomatosis, 73, 74, 81
Blastomycosis, 19, 22
Chromomycosis, 20, 22
Coccidioidomycosis, 21, 22
Cryptococcosis, 177, 190
Dermatophytosis, 95, 96
Epidermodysplasia verruciformis, 98, 105
Herpes, 110, 115, 270, 272
Kaposi's sarcoma, 76, 81
Leishmaniasis, 180, 190
Lepromatous leprosy, 181, 191
Orf, 101, 106
Myrmecium, 100, 105
Verruca plana, 103, 106
Verruca vulgaris, 104, 106

Inflammatory disorders
Blistering disorders
Bullous pemphigoid, 122, 125, 130
Dermatitis herpetiformis, 126, 130
Herpes gestationis, 125
Porphyria cutanea tarda, 129, 131

Interface reactions
Discoid lupus erythematosus, 86, 92
Erythema multiforme, 269, 272
Fixed drug reaction, 141, 147
Graft-versus-host disease, 142, 147
Lichen nitidus, 143, 147
Lichen planus, 144, 148
Lichen striatus, 145, 148
Pigmented purpuric dermatosis, 134, 136
Pityriasis lichenoides et varioliformis acuta, 146, 148
Porokeratosis, 91, 93

Miscellaneous
Acne keloidalis, 235, 242
Axillary granular parakeratosis, 94, 96
Burn, 268, 272
Chondrodermatitis nodularis helicis, 85, 92

Flegel's disease, 87, 92
Granuloma faciale, 236, 242
Mastocytosis, 138, 140, 239, 243
Nutritional deficiency, 271, 272
Pigmented purpuric dermatosis, 134, 136
Polymorphous light eruption, 128, 131
Porokeratosis, 91, 93
Radiation dermatitis, 265, 266
Scabies, 121, 123
Sweet's syndrome, 241, 243

Panniculitis and other disorders of adipose tissue
Erythema induratum, 163, 171
Erythema nodosum, 164, 171
Lipodermatosclerosis, 165, 172
Lupus profundus, 166, 172
Pancreatic fat necrosis, 167, 172
Polyarteritis nodosa, 168, 173
Subcutaneous fat necrosis of the newborn, 169, 173
Subcutaneous T-cell lymphoma, 170, 173

Papulosquamous disorders
Pityriasis rubra pilaris, 90, 93
Psoriasis, 17, 18
Inflammatory linear verrucous epidermal nevus, 88, 92

Spongiotic disorders
Arthropod bite reaction, 118, 122
Eosinophilic spongiosis, 117–123
Pityriasis rosea, 135, 136
Stasis dermatitis, 78, 82

Vasculitis
Erythema induratum, 163, 171
Granuloma faciale, 236, 242
Leukocytoclastic vasculitis, 133, 136
Polyarteritis nodosa, 168, 173

Malformations
Accessory digit, 3, 7
Accessory nipple, 4, 7
Accessory tragus, 5, 7
Auricular pseudocyst, 41, 49
Branchial cleft cyst, 42, 49
Cutaneous endometriosis, 44, 50
Dermoid cyst, 45, 50

Malignant tumors
Carcinomas
Adenoid cystic carcinoma, 66, 69
Aggressive digital papillary adenocarcinoma, 59, 64
Basal cell carcinoma, morpheaform, 55, 58
Bowen's disease, 15, 18
Merkel cell carcinoma, 228, 233
Metastatic breast carcinoma, 53, 57
Microcystic adnexal carcinoma, 54, 57
Mucinous carcinoma, 245, 247
Paget's disease, 102, 106
Proliferating pilar tumor, 261, 263

Melanocytic tumors
Melanoma, 196, 201
Melanoma, balloon cell, 183, 191
Melanoma, desmoplastic, 197, 201

Miscellaneous
Atypical fibroxanthoma, 216, 223
Dermatofibrosarcoma protuberans, 205, 213
Langerhans cell histiocytosis, 137, 140
Leukemia (myelogenous), 237, 242
Lymphoma, 238, 242
Mycosis fungoides, 139, 140
Myeloma, 240, 243
Renal cell carcinoma, 185, 192
Subcutaneous T-cell lymphoma, 170, 173

Vascular tumors
Angiosarcoma, 72, 80